HUMANS ARE FUCKED

Critical Science, Hapless Humor, Hopeless Behavior, Then: Climate Change Consequences

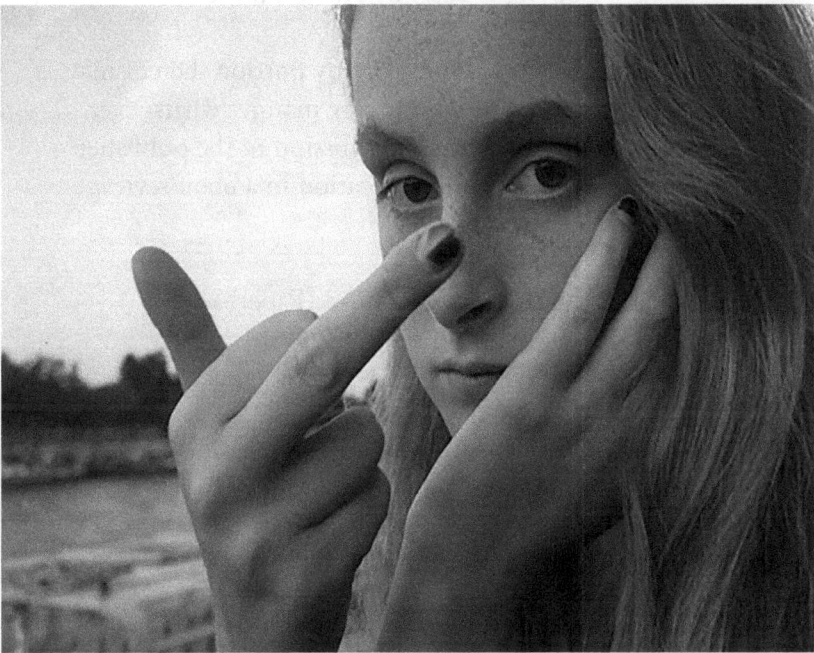

"You are killing my planet. Why must you?"

DAVID HAWK

ISBN 978-1-962363-30-3 (Paperback)
ISBN 978-1-962363-32-7 (Hardcover)
ISBN 978-1-962363-31-0 (Ebook)

Inquiries and Book Orders should be addressed to:

Leavitt Peak Press
17901 Pioneer Blvd Ste L #298, Artesia, California 90701
Phone #: 2092191548

CONTENTS

PREFACE

YOUTH WILL ENCOUNTER
UNPLEASANT FUTURES

Dedicated to the world's youth, those experiencing ever greater challenges to continuance of life. These contents discuss that continuance relative to instabilities created by humans, and how such is expanding beyond human ability to manage. I'm sorry.

Business as usual continuation poses serious threats to the context of life. Life requires well-being nurtured by a natural environment. Humans seem to reject this truism. They work to expand the bringing of turbulence into their context. Even when it is widely known that life depends on a healthy environment most humans remain firmly seated in front of this era's sources of hopelessness: 2-D restricting computers and/or TV images of all that is from 1-D thinking of digital differences.

The current situation for humans is not new. It has evolved over two centuries via reliance on mechanically unfortunate metaphors, machines, and methods, all designed to consume and destroy context. As such, humans have come to destroy much of the natural context while knowing it is essential to life's continuance. Somehow humans diligently work to create piles of seemingly purposeful trash to put in and on the earth, as well as to float in the oceans.

Standing on a trash-economy humans arrogantly describe their work as "Superior to Nature." Science tells us that we were and are wrong in this and will pay a price for such thinking. Biblical writings were not right. Yes, the results enrich a few but at a cost to the many and consequences for the context of it all. The lack of distribution of wealth resulting from what humans call work needs to be reconsidered. Its results need to be diversified and distributed in a manner similar to the basis of healthy plant life. Diversity enriches life but the human perspective clearly opposes this. In its limits to life it is simply wrong resulting in an uneconomic economy of shameful results for most humans and much of nature. There seem to be serious limits to being human based on human thinking.

> "History is for human self-knowledge...the only clue to what man can do is what man has done. The value of history, then, is that it teaches us what man has done and thus what man is."[1]

Application of societal principles mostly demonstrates no principles. Going deeper into regulations we see societal regulations as a major descriptor of law enforcement principles for men to achieve, which they don't, or can't. The formation of laws relies on differences that make no difference for finding the good. Legalities mostly become societal low points, and illustrate use of differences such as skin color, cultural background, male/female sex, and ownership of property. Valuation based on piles of dirt and its ownership is included in much of what we call regulation. Much is made of trivial differences, in that they make no difference to life, but great difference to administration of laws.

The above encourages citizens to fall back from challenges to life and say: "Its tough out there. That is why I'll stay in here." As such allowing those with wealth to set the masculine over the feminine, company owners over workers, and strategic thinkers over honest actors and thus emphasize differences that sow discord thus keeping corrupt leadership in power. Rule systems like "divide and conquer" become standard to retention of wrongfully granted power. Thus, there is little energy left for improving life absent staged hierarchy. Thus, the hierarchy remains and the differences in wealth and power grow.

---

[1] R.G. Collingwood, *The Idea of History*, England: Oxford Press, 1946.

At the Stockholm School of Economics, we would say, "Remember, that the Nobel Prize in Economics is not based on science, or truth." Economics mostly concentrates on collecting, not sharing, or dividing, empires of dirt. Such is in urgent need of change. Herein we will challenge the status quo and widespread acceptance of its problems via introduction of the *entropic process*. Thus, the most universal law of the universe becomes the ultimate manager of human affairs. The entropic end state ends in the simple burying of former life in a pile of dirt. Later the family, friends and enemies gather to divide piles of dirt with greater economic value.

In 1965 an Australian, Fred Emery, combined with a Scottish Researcher, Eric Trist, in describing the end state for business as usual. They described how limits on human intelligence and behavior were creating a turbulent environment.[2] I took their thesis further to show how it would deteriorate what was crucial for life and endanger life beyond instabilities. They described how the accepted versions of economics between humans were bringing instability to life's context. Associated with this the social systems were being led into instability, a condition that was counter to requirements of systems of life. Their concern was as important as was the disregard shown upon its publication.

Management researchers had no interest in what Emery and Trist were talking about. They accused Emery and Trist of emphasizing doom and gloom about business as usual, and such was counterproductive to the human future. They argued adding additional optimism to business as usual, where it remained strong in boardrooms and classrooms. Key was the question: "Even if the Emery and Trist thesis was true why must they present it in such a negative light?" Regardless, most business researchers ignored the discussion and kept on doing the usual via concern for productivity improvements via business as usual.

---

[2]   Fred Emery and Eric Trist, "The causal texture of organizational environment," *Human Relations*, Volume 18, Issue 1, London: Tavistock Publications, Feb. 1965. (Eric, advisor to my climate change dissertation research.)

Dark clouds of change in the context of business now approach. Turbulence of the seventies and eighties became more pronounced. Back then energy flows came to be restrictive. Now it's different. Energy demand generates inflation. While business as usual continues in schools and journals its status is being changed. A rapidly growing contingent of researchers now find merit in the Emery and Trist warning. Noteworthy is how, after agreeing with the early signs of turbulence, those cutting-edge researchers did not seek to calm the environment. Instead, they turned their attention to cybernetics, digitization, and artificial intelligence from their believing humans required technical assistance. Growing threats to life, as noted by Emery and Trist continued and greatly expanded. That situation is now well beyond prior forecast. Life will be grim for occupants of the 21st Century..

Economic models giving emphasis to the technological over the social continue to be favored. Perhaps such is sent to support the God of productivity instead of calming the instability in the natural context. Widespread destruction of nature continues. Even the troubles forecast in the "Tragedy of the Commons" back in 1968 seem calm in contrast to today's surrounding reality.

Concern for potential termination of planetary life is largely ignored while renewed marketing campaigns for expanded economic growth become emphasized. Economic development is outlined as a major passageway to peace and harmony between humans, as well as humans and nature. The argument states that continuous economic growth will soften the anger seen as natural in competing differences.[3] Yes, this seems a bit hopeless, doesn't it?

Humans have long relied on dreams of reason as verbalized by leadership, even if it comes from the mouths of dishonest men, men whose passion for positions of power reigns supreme regardless of costs to who and whatever. Bio and psycho threats are more real each day, but economists pay little attention to such. The pattern contin-

---

[3]   Joel N. Shurkin, *True Genius: The Live and Work of Richard Garwin, The most Influential Scientist you've never heard of,* New York: Prometheus Books, 2017, (Richard, a friend who helped me organize conferences on war.)

ues. They ignore their role in environmental catastrophes, especially those generated by human leadership.

Herein I will argue for experimentation with the counterweight of hollow hope. Called hopelessness, it shifts attention to the ugly downside of leadership. Then we can ask: Why do humans accept the worst characteristics of humans in their leaders? Why is moral absence common among leaders?

Bad leadership consequences are herein called leadershit. They are grim, but somehow are given and retain power over others. They are seen to continually spread lies herein called the shoveling of shit. Leadershit mostly ends as unfortunate upon the unfortunate. Then, many ask: Don't those who follow deserve what they follow, thus receive? Perhaps they do, but such is not our focus herein. Important to this book is understanding how a societal group comes to generate and adhere to lies. In response I will argue for the use of an unusual concept, one I believe to be key to warning us that we are wrong. It concentrates on a concept used extensively under other titles, but here is called *negative entropy*. It is like a large human dream boat, about to sink. Once you place your trust in such the obvious lies streaming out from it seem trivial, even unbelievable. The dream boat is leaking and listing.

Negative entropy defies the laws of physics. It simply cannot exist in our universe. None-the-less much in human affairs presumes it does exist and/or that humans will soon discover it via our intellectual powers. It is key to marketing schemes, especially those translated for wider public use via advertising. Our human highway to hell seems paved by negative entropy. We can see how it is responsible for many acts ending in climate change consequences. Believing in finding negentropy is a road to happiness that ensures finding the unhappiness of climate change. Perhaps this explains why humans come to seek such unfortunate forms of leadership.

If you are unsure of this just turn on your TV, or turn up its volume, and reflect on the essential message in product and/or campaign commercials. Look carefully at those images attempting to make you happy, even if you know they aren't true. But, if you listen too long, and reflect too deeply, you might come to realize that marketing and its sinister sister, advertising, are intolerable to societal improvement. You watch the selling of negative entropy while in search of happiness.

If this seems confusing, look into Celine's "Death on the Installment Plan." He describes the false selling of negative entropy as key to attracting money from the uninformed (i.e., dumb) in what he hopes to be a successful scam. His book is in tragic humor prose. To avoid the humor but see the tragic look of scientists attempting what Celine suggest please look at Ludwig Boltzmann as explained in books by Arieh Ben-Naim.

Based on the above I propose we experiment with abandoning those false promises underlying hope from lies relative to negentropy. To do this, we can look at the hopelessness underlying the hope as presented by bad leadership. We can thus go deeper into the human dilemmas presented in Plato's "Allegory of the Cave." His cave is now updated where humans act to collect the resources required of the industrial. Using cave metaphors we can look at coal mines in the United States, Russia, Europe, and China. Coal mines offered optimistic sources of energy from digging up hope of progress. Sadly, this became a primary source of CO_2 creating climate change that would end life. As in Plato's Cave, many humans avoid leaving their caves to seek change.

Consistent with the above, humans spent ten thousand years removing raw materials from nature in support of producing products of whatever in ever more productive and anti-natural ways. Productivity mattered more than products. During the last two hundred years the rate of resource removals has expanded exponentially. This continues as a threat to life via its consequences.

In 2020 the situation became serious. Via CO_2 accumulation climate change consequences began to be experienced. Key were concerns with: 1) did humans realize that future debts had been accruing from prior short-term gains, then, 2) did they care, and/or 3) did humans continue to presume they were sufficiently superior to all that there was no reason to care?

These questions provide clues to current efforts to design a new way of living, one that is less obedient to entropy while dreaming about the efficiency of inefficient use of natural materials and energies to create meaningless products and lifestyles. Please note that in 1856 a female scientist came out against this and warned scientists of the consequences of a CO2 buildup from industry burning coal. Then, the masculine weakness rose to specifically disregard her research and ignore her concerns for the planet.

It is now clearly too late to avoid the late term consequences from industrialization. Threats from nature are now growing and expanding. They seem to bring systemic instability that greatly threatens life. Early on we will see economic wreckage begin in the systemic elimination of the insurance industry. This will happen due to the expanding climate hazards to objects of insurance. Following this the mortgage industry will begin to close, as insurance for the mortgage is essential. Provision of shelter will become impossible. The next stage downward will be a significant reduction of tax money from real estate, funds used to keep citizens safe, secure, and educated.

As climate stability disappears, we will hear about the need for a new and stronger kind of leadership. This will worsen the social dimension of climate change. Herein I argue for adaptation of the hunting-party model of old, where leadership was kept fluid, like the situations in which it is used. The leader at a particular time was the most competent in the skill needed at the time. It was like self-governance arising from collaborations, not cheap and easy authoritarian orders overall, no matter the situation. Just now we seem to be going towards an ever more authoritarian-based centralization of power, but this will not help manage climate change's consequences. Reliance of power from the tradition of mobilizing hate towards differences, all to organize followers, is as Hitler did for Germany and Trump now attempts for renewing America. Such always arrives at a bad ending for humans involved. The Hunting Party model, as developed by Gunnar Hedlund and I, and described by Tom Peters in his editorials, offers a sounder pathway for leadership during growth of network form organizations, as in IT. Yes, it opposes the religious tradition of hierarchical forms. Hierarchical approaches rely on the many listening to the few, where the few are often seen to be incompetent.

A central concern behind this book is helping citizens become capable of discerning the fundamental differences between leadership and leadershit. Most leaders after 1850 had a shortage of what is needed today. Most leaders continue to be seen as too expensive to keep around. Change is urgently needed. The cost associated with wrong leaders during the next fifty years will likely grow. A new definition of leadership is needed to give emphasis to those having competence in understanding context. In addition, leaders need to go light on their emphasis with egocentricity of self.

The costs from a bad episode in history are mounting, and overdue. Key to characterizing from where the cost of two centuries of abuse arises is to call attention to processes of industrialization. No one thought it would become so anti-natural and so very expensive to continuance of life, but it became so. Nature now responds to that unprovoked war by foreclosing many human operations based on the industrial method. Nature's options for such can have many names. Climate change is a major one, where its consequences become opposite to conditions needed to maintain life, but there are other issues.

History illustrates that some bad humans have managed to become leaders, then had long runs doing harm to many. Metaphorically speaking we might say leadership has now brought humans to bankruptcy. Key traits of such are egocentricity, arrogance about humans, and collecting their share of short-term gain while ignoring all cost associated with long-term pain.

The world's youth see the evidence of all this and find it upsetting. They hear rules for what they must do and must not do each day, yet such directives are trivial in light of what leaders do and don't do. Youth feel disheartened, then walk away in disbelief. Most important is how they are educated to shut up, to resist seeing weakness in leaders while avoiding change. In schools they are thus encouraged to memorize answers and avoid asking questions. Those answers are how we got into trouble. The important questions have yet to be asked. Youth see clear parallels between change and nature, then ask how we can pretend to not change. They ask adults to explain how changelessness fits with an apparent arrival of ever more violently behaving climate change. When they comment on the consequences of such they are advised by "leaders" to:

> "Go to sleep my child. The climate has always been changing, and what changes is logically no longer there to talk about. Reality, as we know and like it, is changelessness, i.e., It never changes." [4]

Tradition is carefully wrapped up in culture via changelessness. How can this work during drastically unpredictable change. It can't. To deny change under such conditions becomes a denial of life. Yes, we can become rich marketing a non-cents changelessness and then promising the products so produced will never need maintenance or repairs. Such Ads now seem ever more trivial with time. At times we sense that it is all nonsense but when selling slows we move down to an even lower form of nonsense to support business as usual. Meanwhile, the negative consequences become ever more dangerous, ending in no business.

A pattern of technological advancement can be seen in expanding business as usual. Conflicted humans, where the number of these is rapidly growing, are seen to evolve. They begin in simple unpleasantness, move into anger, pull out knives, and then turn to a technological upgrade of guns. When this fails to work out we dream of using nuclear bombs. The situation is related in our responses to climate change consequences. We see contextual devastation in death defining temperatures, then extreme droughts, never before experienced floods, and starvation encouraging mass migration. This will defy long-standing promises from cultures to human occupants that there will be continuous improvement at home if they follow rules of diligent work and obedience to governance. Such now appears vacuous and mass migration will upset those promised stable wealth.

---

[4] David Hawk, dissertation, 1979. Parmenides, then Plato, argued reality is changelessness. Heraclitus, a troublemaker, argued the opposite – change was essential to life. 6th Century BC

INTRODUCTION

1. Changelessness Wrapped in Culture

As culture emerged in society it offered an initial promise - to support and encourage humans to adopt a changeless philosophy. In this way, lacking change agents and the problems associated with seeing a future, humans could focus on getting short-term gains from non-changing surroundings. Where necessary the problems associated with change could then be settled later, and humans could pay up later. Perhaps they could even arrange for others to pay off their debts or rise above future problems from change by emphasizing technological advancement. With technology humans could become insulated from change and isolated from its uncertainties.

To pretend changelessness often relies on artful lying during face-to-face encounters. Just now deceit is aided by humanly developed AI technology. Computer technology and AI began with considerable limits from using Aristotle's thinking for design of digital communication. It was based on the twosomes of either/or as found in 0/1 choices. Some humans found this far too artificial and moved on to seek greater capabilities as seen in natural communication. This has led to newer AI models, ones designed to help humans communicate with others and self, while being able to pretend the strength of being clearly natural. When I'm asked about the impact of Artificial Intelligence I usually comment: "Why not, let's just hope it's more intelligent than humans were."

To help you see the content problems in face-to-face, as well as from behind communication, and see what AI will do about them, you might look in two books. The first, from 1975, is a John Brunner book titled *The Shockwave rider.* It was about the introduction of a future that Bruner thought was best avoided. The hero removes Congress, replacing them with AI. This is because Congress was seen as very slow in dealing with the President. AI could relate immediately with the President's wishes as authoritarian. Upon seeing the results the book's hero bails out, removes his identity, and hides in nature.

A second book comes from the work of Professor Harry Frankfurt in 2005, as printed by Princeton University Press under the title of: "*On Bullshit.*" Therein he discusses something much scarier than lies, that he calls bullshit, or a system of lies, much like how some leading-edge politicians talk. Understanding Frankfurt's definition of bullshit is also useful to better understand economic theories, such as that of Adam Smith. If you have read Smith's work, you might recall his emphasis on a glorious rationale for freedom from want. Such is accessible via economic exchange where that exchange come from resources of "natural capital" as found in those "renewable raw materials." Such can go round and round in economically applied cycles. His dream came to be proven wrong in the 1850-56 period via the clarification of the laws of thermodynamics.

Renewable raw materials never existed, nor were ever created by projects in science. Thus, Smith's version of economics was and is truly based on "bullshit." This may be why so many humans understood it and became attracted to it and thus structured their lives around it. The Smith theory is even used in gaining more funding of a science project. This is seen when a research group needs additional funding every few years on a thermodynamics project. The group begins with a press release describing how they are on the edge of a major discovery of negative entropy. As such, they must have more funding to get to their target.

Smith's proposition of March 9, 1776, was and continues to be very attractive, it's just that it cannot be true. His followers often say, if only we could find a way to restore those resources required for economic production. They are needed in the products humans consume. If there was no waste, then everything would be great. In my research this is classified under the heading of the quest for finding "negative entropy." It's interesting in that about 95% of humans are passionate in believing such will be found or always existed.

When you build chariots for others to buy, you should avoid mentioning that maintenance will be needed to continue their use, or it will become garbage. In 1850-56 the carefully articulated laws of thermodynamics helped explain why negentropy was and would always be impossible. If Smith were still with us, he would be able to see the garbage continuing to pile up in his recycling piles. Economic-minded humans continue to invest much in marketing Smith and negentropy. They imply humans will finally discover how the laws of thermodynamics will be overturned. They also write articles on how climate change consequences from entropy will then be avoided on the planet. From this human can continue with their search for human happiness. They can then go out and acquire those forever-larger SUVs. No problem as the manufacturer talks of someday recycling it. Such was and continues to be key to business as usual. The youth can change all this if it's not too late.

Smith's idea of creating human lust in economic exchange comes out from a shallow and widespread human dream, one that grows more expensive with time. It is a belief that we humans can do things to bring benefit to themselves, and there will be no cost to them or any earthly context. Industrialization thus sent that dream on a two-hundred-year rampage based on the idea of negentropy.

Einstein, Hawkings, and Carl Sagan were very clear that Smith's thinking was a problem that leads to other larger problems. Most who mention this get criticized by that 95% who are passionate about finding negentropy. Carl Sagan critiqued such but was pretty soft about it. It looked like a side issue to his emphasis on the cosmos, or so he told me. Thus, most were not upset with his pessimism about the role of entropy in the human future. Most of his followers skipped over it in thinking of the glory of human conquest of other worlds, just like in the movies.

Nicholas Georgescu-Roegen, on the other hand, focused on the role entropy played in human and cosmic existence. In 1971 he described how entropy overrode economics, especially Smith's approach to it. He talked of humans fading into nothingness via entropy eating economics. Georgescu-Roegen's clarity, as well as his criticism of business-as-usual, set him up for much anger and no rewards. He was seen as a hopeless pessimist, except by Schumpeter, who said he was the most promising economist of the 20th Century. By 2050 he may be the last economist worthy of understanding.

Georgescu-Rogen described how those privatized short-term economic gains will come to be buried under a deteriorated natural context. He reminds us that such a context, not recyclable, is what life is dependent upon. Smith's focus was on continual motivation of humans to acquire ever more dollars, even where acquiring them made little sense (cents?). Such could be used to encourage billionaires in 2024 to balloon their individualized arrogance while ignoring the cost of a deteriorated context. If things get too challenging, they can buy a space trip to another more hospitable planet. They continue to be attracted to Smith's values where only one value matters, that of their private bank account. Youth will move on from this shallow thinking to seek a noteworthy future not built on the marketing of negentropy. Business as usual will have gone out of business by then.

The problem with introducing change can be seen in recent marketeering by Mike Huckabee via his "truth telling for youth." His comments are consistent with the 95% and raises the flag to those saying: "the climate has always been changing, so what?"[5] Youth will undoubtedly become angry with the Huckabee advisement as reality intrudes on Huckabee's advertisement. Related to this is a rule of humans in how to know and/or find out what you don't know. It's a method. It comes from a Greek tradition of humans seeking the causes of it all, including themselves.

---

[5]   Keerti Gopal, *Inside Climate News*, "Mike Huckabee's 'Kids Guide to the Truth About Climate Change' Shows the Changing Landscape of Climate Denial." July 3`, 2023.

2. Cause-Effect Logic: It's Weaknesses

Cause-effect logic has been a centerpiece of human affairs and the building of a knowledgebase from which to know that we call science. When humans face a bothersome situation, they search for its cause. For example, your wife wishes to divorce you. What caused this? Was it what you said to her this morning, or you hitting her last night when she commented on how small you were? Finally, from careful examination of all possible causes you discover the cause of the problem is simply her. From this you begin to feel better, but only temporarily. Yes, it is nice to feel good, even temporarily, but during our management of the cause we find reality to be different. We see how our use of cause-effect thinking ends up worsening the initial problems, so much so that finding the cause may well become "the cause" of many problems. Youth will need to see this to better understand why life as more natural is more interesting than what can be seen as cause-effect relations. To begin with we might first look at the concept of management, then begin to note how our limitations and problems often begin and end with the first three letters of the concept of management. We need to do better.

Key to understanding all this we should examine the leadership behind it and qualities of such. Perhaps leadership is a misnomer. Its results have the smell of leadershit. Upon interviewing adults, you will ask: "How can leaders be those in society with nowhere to go?" Some youths have already turned from the hopelessness on the horizon to seek new ways to un-fuck what has so clearly been fucked. While most leaders in education and many in business think business as usual needs to be tightened, a few special business CEOs are urgently seeking business as unusual prior to no business being there.

Business as unusual requires rejection of hateful leaders who long wandered around seeming to have no place to go. Via the WSJ many were proud of their nothingness. With no concern for direction, they are seen to turn against those around them. To have followers was all that mattered. Leaders such as Putin, Trump, or Musk are examples to other lesser beings, just as lesser beings from the past inspired them to adopt Ayn Rand feelings for life. Emphasize was and is on servicing self, seeing nature as an obstacle, and harshly criticizing those who dare sound, smell, look, and act better than they. As Bierce defined it in 1883.

> "Egotist, n. A person of low taste, more interested in himself than in me."[6]

Yes, many attracted to becoming leaders are of such quality. Such is an important aspect of why our organizations are so out of touch with the ever more rapidly descending phenomenon of climate change. They are more interested in their "in here" than in the "out there." Now to escape from the contemporary model of a president, CEO, father, etc.? I would advise, as I did to China's Expert Council in Feb. 2007 as they were preparing to select new leadership for China, move on from the egoist Leader issue, as embraced by Confucius teachings to the sincere advice that opposed such in 6th Century BC teachings of Lao Tzu.

> "A leader is best when people barely know he exists, when his work is done, his aim fulfilled, they will say: we did it ourselves."

It's hard to emphasize such leadership qualities, especially if they are successful. Leadership power, as measured by items like salary, forcefully rejects ideas of Lao Tzu. This is seen in schools and places of work. Herein emphasis is on the consequences of climate change. Primary in generating and managing such acts of weak men standing behind strong arrogance, all in search of their immortality. These men support the authoritarian posture where they eagerly take advantage of others and their context for their selfish ends. If asked about relations to nature they ask what that is, then as they get up to leave, they offer love and prayers for your sadness.

A related and equally important trait of such humans is that they presume humans will locate access to immortality via discovery of negative entropy. Yes, they also hope they will be the one to secure

---

[6]   Ambrose Bierce, *The Devil's Dictionary*, New York: Hill and Wang, 1957, p. 42.

its patten, not their neighbors. Immortality has long been key desire of weak men. Not only will climate change concerns become irrelevant, but humans will find an immortality technology.

It is also important to note that these men are also seen to carry a special attitude towards women as non-men, born to serve men. This was illustrated long ago in the Garden of Eden story. Shallow men find management of the female is easier when women are in the depths of despair as seen in the intention of the American Comstock Act of 1873. It remains in force. (It banned use of words such as fuck and women discussing birth control with each other.)

Even if you disagree with the tone of the above comments it is increasingly difficult to ignore that such bad leadership and management has brought destruction to the natural world, and those depending on it for life. The gain for this loss was industrial production to meet psycho-wants of sad humans. We have now evolved to access these wants via constant 2-D computer imaging while under the management of 1-D politics of a single line with an opposing point at each end. We seldom reflect on 4-D mortality over time nor 5-D existence beyond the limits of materiality. Focusing on our 2-D mobile phone visioning we seldom notice how our nature filled third dimension is governed by 1-D choice for turning left or right at the next intersection. Via the limits of such we work to destroy mother nature's developments experienced in 3D.

Returning to the Adam Smith limitations for economics, we find we are not at a very complementary stage for the conduct of political debates and choices in a group. We somehow have come to presume that money is part of political choice, and we best tolerate it, but we seldom go deeper. Unfortunately, the role of economics and money is great. We pay much for tolerating purchase of politics. With money allowed in the system we can restrict political choices and bad laws. This is seen throughout the US Court System. Recent numbers from political science researchers Jeffrey Winters and Benjamin Page point this out:

> "…each of the top 400 or so richest Americans has on average about 22,000 times the political power of the average

member of the bottom 90 percent, and each of the top 100 or so had nearly 60,000 times as much."[7]

During the Covid crisis the 700 American billionaires collected another $2 trillion for their collective war chests, amounting to almost $3 billion more for each billionaire. Of course, part of these additions were given to the political campaigns to win elections and arrive at regulations and tax reliefs of benefit to billionaires. In conclusion management is the problem with emphasis on the weakness in the first three letters of the concept. As such the masculine became an ally of the entropic process. As will be discussed later, entropy governs father time's 4th dimension death sentences placed upon all life. As such, male activities speed the decay, disintegration, and death process in life, especially to the natural environment.[8]

The clearest sign of stupidity creating hopelessness is seen in what we call defense. Therein anti-life weapon systems move the larger context ever closer to destruction while making some billionaires even richer. The rich become richer, the poor become more scared, and the environment disintegrates towards death.[9]

We defuse our fear and ignorance while shopping to have what we didn't want and need. Thus buy an ever-larger SUVs to drive around looking for nature. If we find such we wonder if we can do better?

An argument is made herein that the human response to environmental deterioration has worsened and brought about climate change consequences. Much comes from the misallocation of benefits from workers' work thus visible, yet unseen, consequences later

---

[7] Jeffrey Winters and Benjamin Page, "Oligarchy in the United States? Perspectives on Politics," Patrioticmillionaires.org, July 29, 2023.

[8] If you want to see more about the activities of those arguing for negative entropy to be invented look at scientists of July 2023 using "Superconductivity Claims" to attract more research funding every few years.

[9] In 1986 a friend and I staged a symposium at New Jersey Institute of Technology around Richard Garwin, co-designer of the nuclear bomb to discuss the future of this process. A major two-day event for NJIT students, about twenty speakers attended, including President Reagan's Head of Start Talks and the Soviet Ambassador to the UN.

appear. The two need to be dealt with as an integrated set. The argument then goes further and deeper.

3. Negentropy: Key to Climate Change Consequences

We have now arrived at one of the most fundamental difficulties in being humans. It is known as entropy and assumes the central role in climate change consequences arriving in life. To respond we hold wide beliefs in negative entropy. While entropy of the rule of the universe and not to be avoiding in our actions on earth we tend to ignore it. Instead, we turn to activities that represent "negative entropy" in what we do. It is also an effective way to obscure the reality of "entropy."

Negentropy is a doorway to the dream existence with immortality awaiting us. Disheartening to me is how tightly connected business education is to reliance on negative entropy discourse, especially that in the teaching of marketing and its ugly sister advertising.

Ads provide the means for billionaires to attract more resources, humans being attracted to more shopping and thus consequences of climate change. Herein I will show how sad this is in that neg-entropy does not and will exist in our universe. Negentropy is the greatest of lies yet is the one that perhaps 95% of humans want to and need to thus believe. With such we can discard the death certificate issued with our birth certificate.

Much will be said herein about negentropy being the key to why and how human's fuck themselves, and thus the life on our earth. This returns us to the importance of *leadership* qualities. In addition to relying on marketing of *negative entropy* current leaders in government and business rely on what we shall call "cause-effect" logic. This comes from Aristotle's digital divide sponsoring the design of early computerization. Therein we found axioms for students to worship the bi-polar twosome. This came from and reinforced the limitations in seeing how effects begin in causes. As such causes become the basic tools for management of individuals, organizations, and the planet. Based on extensive research I now take great issue with the model of managing reality. It has created a new model of reality, one that is not manageable.

Herein I will argue for moving to a model of seeing how *effects arise from prior effects* in an evolutionary change process, not from causes that can be isolated and boxed, as many dangerously outdated books on the science as changelessness argue. Via many research projects I came to distance myself from the value of cause-effect logic, as well as digital modeling of the situation attempting to be understood. In a joint lecture in 1980 with my late friend Carl Sagan he addressed this limitation of human thought. He wrote about such later in one of his books.

> "The Second Law of Thermodynamics states that in the Universe as a whole, disorder increases as time goes on. (Of course, locally worlds and life and intelligence can emerge, at the cost of a decrease in order elsewhere in the Universe.) But if we live in a Universe in which the present Big Bang expansion will slow, stop, and be replaced by a contraction, might the Second Law then be reversed? Can effects precede causes?"[10]

4. Management and Leadershit

Many will come t realize the value in becoming a life-long student of reality by questioning most societal rules. This is greatly helped via the reading of the important books of society. With that in mind I offer an 18-page annotated book list in the appendix. This was mostly composed by past students during many years. They found the books listed interesting and helpful. The same students composed the following diagram to depict business as usual.

---

[10] Carl Sagan, The Demon-Haunted World: Science As A Candle In The Dark, New York: Ballantine Books, 1997. P. 332

Normal Problem-Solving Flows

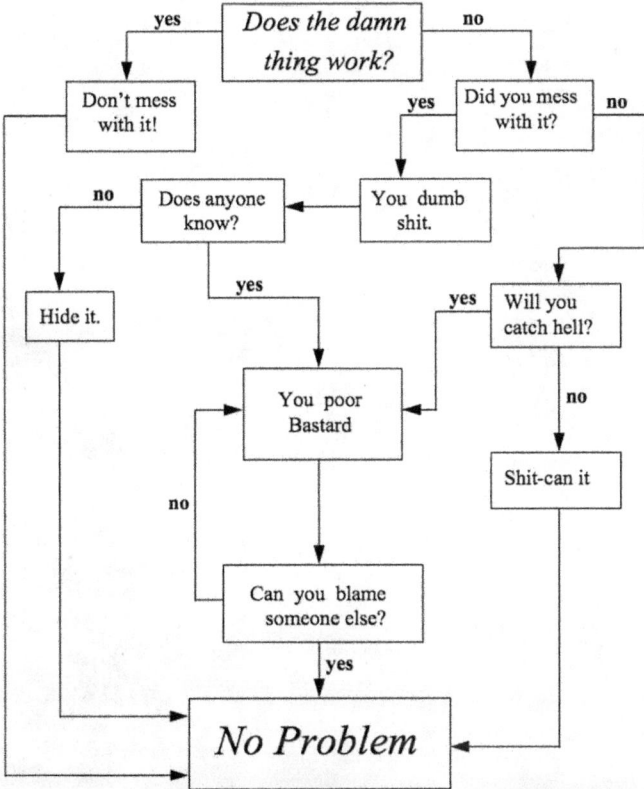

Source: Unknown

We might call this the Elon Musk, Donald Trump diagram for success where shit wins. Since, per the diagram, leaders never make mistakes, and followers can be mistaken it is thus key for leaders to focus on grabbing credit for whatever goes well while tossing shit at those below them. It all works in the organization as those below on the hierarchy of power are disallowed from any complaining or criticism of what comes from above, Bible included.

I

APPROACHING AN END-STATE

This is not a book of entertainment. The contents bring attention to a dire situation on a changing planet, then explains why and how you must change. You, your family, and colleagues will need to change what you value in your life and especially in your activities that define how you relate to continuance of humans and life on this planet. Key will be modification of your economic thinking. It begins in questioning your role in supporting a religion known as industrialization. This is steeped in "Banking on Short-Term Gains while avoiding thoughts of the Long-Term Pains that approach." An earlier book was written under a similar title, but most humans were buried under challenges of the short-term. They mostly disregarded the concern for when and who would pay the debt, now called climate change. Most of those who even noticed such was on their horizon felt the long-term costs and issues would be resolved via new technologies and techniques.

On the back cover of that book there is a quote related to the evolution of human values. It's from Leonard Cohen's last album prior his death and says: "As he died to make men holy. Let us die to make things cheap." Cohen felt we should consider reversing our values about the future. He saw practices in business as usual to be troublesome. Herein I will argue for experimentation with business as unusual. The ten-thousand-year track-record of humans arriving to now is not reassuring.

Humans seeking reality on 2-D screens is troublesome. The normal seems ever more disheartening from seeing 2-D based on 1-D thinking and 0-D politics. The contents that follow attempt to explain some of this then offer advice on where humans might look to find questions that can lead to a better future and adopt values for creating it. The alternative seems certain to illustrate what it means to be fucked. Related to this human history is recorded as a "fight against shit." Record of the rudiments in North and South America, Africa, Asia, and Europe mostly illustrate the cost of bad leadership allowed within arrogant humanism. From this there is little hope for finding a better future.

A "better" path to a better place will need to rise above past caricatures of leadership by those who have nowhere to go, then watching such leadership become leadershit. The Greeks taught that self-governance is the ideal but based on what they experienced such was not possible for humans to access. They then drifted to ideas of democracy which they pointed out as a miserable approach to governance but the best available to humans. As democracy seems to be losing its attraction to most in our world we must design something capable of managing today's challenges. Failing in this the chances are great that we will slide down into a low-level autocratic application of hierarchy that assures access to an unfortunate and ugly end-state. Humans are facing very dire characteristics of a context that will not nurture life. Humans created this situation. Can they create a pathway out from it?

1. Imagining the Problem

Clouds from ominous intentions are approaching. They promise serious dangers to life. Appearing as natural, in a sarcastic manner, they pose a darkly ominous nature. They threaten the physical existence of life as we know it, including our need to find clean air, clear water, healthy food, extensive vegetation, and inspiring images without trash.

The sky grows darker each day in ways we have never seen or felt before. Something is quite wrong. Those drawn to science reports know of the approaching conditions and how destructive they will be to what we know to be essential to life. Conditions that exterminate planetary life are rare. It has been several million years since life last dealt with such challenges where 75 to 95% of life was erased prior to again taking hold and expanding. Science points out that there were five prior episodes where much of life was removed from the planet.

I offer small quotations from three recent books that give a sense of the growing concern for life.

1. **Elizabeth Kolbert** outlined the antinatural history of humans in her 2014 book:

    Over the last half billion years there have been five major mass extinctions, when the diversity of life on earth suddenly and dramatically contracted. Scientists are currently monitoring the sixth extinction, predicted to be the most devastating since the asteroid impact that wiped out the dinosaurs. This time around, the cataclysm is us.[11]

2. **David Wallace-Wells** offered greater clarity in 2019 from five additional years of research on the same issue. He describes how life will leave via conditions of global warming.

    It is worse, much worse, than you think. The slowness of climate change is a fairy tale, perhaps as pernicious as the one that says it isn't happening at all, and comes to us bundled with several others in an anthology of comforting delusions: that global warming is an Artic saga, unfolding remotely; that it is strictly a matter of sea level and coastlines, not an enveloping crisis sparing no place and leaving no life undeformed; that it is a crisis of the "natural" world, not the human one; that those two are distinct, and we live today somehow outside or beyond or at the very least

---

[11] Elizabeth Kolbert, *The Sixth Extinction*, New York: Henry Holt and Company, 2014, inside cover.

defended against nature, not inescapably within and literally overwhelmed by it; that wealth can be a reliable shield against the ravages of warming; that the burning of fossil fuels is the price of economic growth; that growth, and the technology it produces, will inevitably engineer a way out of environmental disaster; that there is any analogue to the scare or scope of this threat, in the long span of human history, that might give us confidence in staring it down.[12]

3. **Greta Thunberg** documents summary comments from more than a hundred leading scholars who have long been concerned about climate change. Printed in 2023, it offers a third and increasingly frightful depiction of our current trajectory to a lifeless planet.

    This is the biggest story in the world, and it must be spoken as far and wide as our voices can carry, and much further still.

    It must be told in books and articles, in movies and songs, at breakfast tables, lunch meetings and family gatherings, in lifts, at bus stops and in rural shops. In Schools, boardrooms, and marketplaces. At airports, in gyms and in bars. In the fields, in the warehouses and on the factory floors. At union meetings, political workshops, and football games. In kindergartens and in old people's homes. In hospitals and car-repair shops. On Instagram, TikTok and the evening news. On dusty country roads and in the streets and alleys of our towns and cities.

    The time has come for us to tell this story, and perhaps even change the ending.[13]

---

[12] David Wallace-Wells, *The Uninhabitable Earth, Life After Warming*, New York: Tim Duggan Books, 2020, page 2.

[13] Greta Thunberg, *The Climate Book*, New York: Penguin Press, 2023, back cover.

She arises from Sweden, the country giving essential support to the 1975-77 research carried out while I was with the Stockholm School of Economics. The project was done within the Institute of International Business, established with friends. They were interested in finding improvements to management of human existence via business as unusual. They, and I, felt strongly that it was too late for continuation of 19th Century business as usual. That history simply faced too many shortcomings as based on ideas about hierarchy, taking resources from the nature, and segmented parts of the world fighting over resultant wealth. Concern at the time was growing with regard to the dumping of the unwanted back into someone else's back yards. Greta had gone to great personal cost to question normal behavior of humans. She was in search of strands of happiness connected to a meaningful existence. Her concern was devoted to the well-being of context. Prior to her birth I had conducted a research project in Sweden of her present concerns. The following quotation comes from the 2019 reprint of my 1979 book about the meaning of 1977 research results.

> There was no success in applying the findings of very concerned companies and government people forty years ago. They saw an urgent need to control environmental deterioration resulting from human activities. They helped recommend a new model for regulation. The situation was then fluid, not fixed, and in need of ideas for business as unusual in both private and public organizations. Back then it was shown how deterioration was expanding and efforts to regulate and limit such were turning bad into worse.

> The situation of environmental deterioration can no longer be addressed via expanded research, invention of new technologies or in modifications in meeting human needs and wants in adjustments to the current neo-classical economic model. We have moved beyond those somewhat understood traditional responses. We now face the consequences of greatly expanded environmental deterioration.

It is now culminating in very dire phenomena such as the one only briefly mentioned in the 1977 study called *climate change*. The best information now suggests humans must move from the business-as-usual responses to meeting the very real human bio-needs while completely rethinking the holographic domain of human psych-wants. [14]

2. A Paradox in Being Human

IIB was an unusual Institute of gifted people. It was well-funded by leading organizations with an emphasis on creating business as unusual via experiments with such. They strongly supported the Institute's first research project, on the consequences of environmental deterioration from business ideas, and operations. It was unusual for its time, to say the least. The IIB Board and many companies gave it full support for experimenting with the uncertainties the world was entering.

The founders of the Institute, Drs. Lars Otterbeck, and Gunnar Hedlund have my greatest respect and much love for that which they attempted to create. Ten years after its creation the Financial Times of London did an article on its research concluding it was the World's Foremost Research Center on Business. For years Professors at places like Harvard tried to do joint work with the Stockholm Institute but didn't succeed in gaining much entry until the new leadership in 1996 welcomed them in. From that point the organization became more "normal" and less particular about researching the future. The search for business as unusual was removed.

The 1975-77 research project, IIB's first, came to be titled, "Environmental Protection: Analytic Solutions in Search of Synthetic Problems." We felt the project confronted growing conflict between nations, cultures, peoples, as well as between people and their environments. This was evidenced in growing national investments

---

[14] David Hawk, *Too Early, Too Late, Now what?*, North Carolina: Brilliant Books, 2019, p. vii.

devoting increasing portions of their science and technology to conduct of war, coupled to clear increases in deterioration of the natural world, as well as shortages in essential energy and material needs to continue industry. The lead in this was by governmental and business leadership as trained in 19th Century models of control. Such was seen to be more problematic than helpful.

Behind and beneath emerging difficulties were presumptions arising from two dominant models. For economic exchange the model was based on Adam Smith's beliefs about providing goods and services. Associated with and giving support to incoherent economics was a model of science that was also purposefully fragmented. As with economics, it was to encourage autonomous development of truths that could be privately patented. Reliance on the reductionistic logic of Aristotle further disintegrated the vision of the natural context of humans being human .

As such we saw a funny and counterproductive combinations of Aynn Rand's behavioral ideas used to integrate economics with Darwin interpretation of forces of biological change. Autonomous economics linked to scientific fragmentation left little time to reflect on the destruction of a context on which life depended. From this a two-year research venture began into environmental deterioration and the business management processes driving it.

The study began by reaching out to organizations thought to be the most extreme examples of the emerging problems. This began with Texaco. The Texaco Board agreed to join the work and thus changed their rules thus allowing their staff to join a research project with an academic institution. Seeing this, many other companies asked to join the project. Once twenty major international firms were involved several governments asked to be part of the research on how to better regulate emerging problems in business. Many of the ideas from the project arose from the work of those working on the project. Their work demonstrated that there was hope. At the time we saw hope in the hopelessness of what we studied. Now we see there were many barriers to realizing the hope, more than we imagined.

3. Alarming Findings, Then Nothing But Silence

In 1977 at the end of the Swedish project mentioned above the Chair of the Wharton Educational Program that I had studied with, Russell Ackoff, contacted me. He said he had read the transcript of the presentation of my work by Sweden's Prime Minister to OECD. He then secured the three research volumes as printed by the Stockholm School of Economics. He commented that he thought it was the best dissertation he had ever seen about the world's future. He said it was a perfect example of why the Systems Sciences Program was needed at Wharton and that, as far as he was concerned, it was a dissertation for a PhD in his program. He said I only needed to return to Wharton for a bit, do the closure paperwork, be reviewed by a committee, and then accept Wharton's PhD.

A research project like the 1975 one in Sweden would not have been possible in other places at that time, especially not in America. While at the Wharton School I checked and many faculty and most company leaders were simply uninterested in an environmental project. They had more important things to worry about. Yes, Sweden did have its problems, but it somehow could see larger problems in the context of the world.

It's helpful to note Greta, from Sweden, to see how her personality is key to what we need more of. She simply wanted to find a human culture that could change and move to emphasize what should matter most. The term "fuck" is used herein as consistent with her protesting intended to wake the elderly and include the tears of the youth to emphasize the situation being left by the elderly.

Another explanation of humans not remembering earlier acts as they come to be connected to bad situations the humans find themselves within is seen in a book. It is about the results of consequences of earlier acts being disconnected from the present via language that confuses. We had been warned of this process in 2005 on the language used by bad leadership. The book was written by a Princeton University professor of philosophy. He defined and described a central trait of deficient humans wanting to be leaders of deficient humans agreeing to follow. Activities of shopping, educating, and selecting leaders, all by humans, were pacifiers to dampen concern about humanly generated mistakes. The title *On Bullshit*[15] described extensive work by humans to dampen concern for life and pathways to its extinction. Bullshit was used in language to separate images gone wrong from leadership initiating them. The book was a precursor to Donald Trump walking down that escalator in his NYC building, to seek becoming the US President. It became the Princeton University Bookstore's largest bestseller.

Such makes use of and accompanies many scientific truths. One example was seen in the seventies discussion of climate change as a hoax. Such an "extinction" was inconceivable. To say a threat was a hoax became a helpful way to make those alive come to feel they are doing well, since they were still alive. This was challenged in 2019 via a very unusual movie titled: "Don't Look Up." What is especially interesting is in the final scene there is a depiction of the importance of leadership of the earth's current business and governmental activities and ideas, the ones that created the sad situation.

Key to this book is the 1975-77 research project based on Sweden. Since that time the failure in its reporting is more noteworthy than the project results of the time. Project results appeared in three volumes as printed by the Stockholm School of Economics, IIB. They were widely endorsed by the heads of the participating organizations with hundreds of copies shared with many other organizations, such as US EPA and similar agencies in other nations. Many companies in the industries in the study also asked for copies of the results. The Organization for Economic Cooperation and Development endorsed its circulation along with other research groups. By late 1977 the research results began to encounter barriers and unhappiness, especially focused on the notation of climate change consequences arising from continued failure in control of environmental deterioration. An example was the US EPA.

In 1975 the Director of US EPA offered to help fund the research as it involved evaluation of different approaches to regula-

---

[15] Harry G. Frankfurt, *On Bullshit*, Princeton, and Oxford: Princeton University Press, 2005. Introduction.

tion of environmental deterioration. The research team was skeptical of such support as it had talked with EPA directors. The day the project was launched we received a note from EPA saying they had withdrawn from project support, and funding. Since we had significant funding from others that was not a problem. During the project we received information support from various directors that liked the projects questions. One month after the final reports appeared and were sent to various EPA Regional Offices I received a letter back from the Director of EPA. He pointed out that not only did he not support the conclusions but could not support the model of research used, its reliance on companies being regulated for plant information. He pointed out that he had collected all copies, about thirty, of the three volumes and they were being sent to my Iowa farm address, as EPA had no further use of them, nor of me. He concluded with a summary comment that he would ensure that no US Government money would ever support my research in the future. During my later representation of the National Science Foundation on a National Academy of Sciences project a new Director of EPA changed their policy and funded a 1993 project they asked me to do on establishing "Energy Star Homes."

Regardless, I did consider the above-described project a failure by 1990 in that no beneficial change was happening based on its recommendation. I previously mentioned that in 1977 Russell Ackoff, my Chair at the Wharton School, wanted me to receive a PhD for the three volumes of research findings. I looked into that some months later with my mentor, Professor Eric Trist also of Wharton. He felt the three volumes were fine, but not a dissertation as they posed no thesis for evaluating what humans did, and how they responded to being regulated. During three months I wrote a 250-page thesis on the chances for humans to regulate environmental deterioration before it became irreversible, i.e., when climate change consequences would be too great to manage.

Once submitted Ackoff was not pleased as it contained a chapter on the history of anarchistic approaches to man attempting to relate to nature, and how it sometimes worked well. None-the-less Ackoff did supported the prior three volumes. An expanded committee was called to review the work. They felt the final thesis book, the one for Eric Trist, was very clear but perhaps too clear as it raised many difficult arguments, such as the idea of approaching climate change. For them I rewrote that volume to make it seem ambiguous, kindly thoughtful and requesting more research to be done, to clarify. It then passed.

The Dean of Wharton at the time was not very kind in his review and vowed that such work would never lead to a PhD in his School. The committee disagreed with him. The President of Penn then got involved and supported the work. It finally passed based on agreement that all four volumes would become the dissertation, and not just the final volume on forms of governance in human history, and how they came to relate to nature. To this day only the fourth volume, written in 1978, has ever made it into the University of Pennsylvania Library. The other three, written in 1977, somehow disappeared in transit. Many believe I never received a PhD based on the controversy surrounding the research.

Climate change was then seen as a hoax and I don't care much about having a PhD, as I never planned on getting one. Relative to climate change consequences another PhD in our world is quite irrelevant. If humans are fucked, and I'm a human, why worry about three initials, as placed after some people's names. Sometimes I get called and referred to as doctor thus I respond with: "Sorry, I'm not a doctor, I have no patients, or patience." Wharton claims I do have a PhD from them.

I outline this story as it continued to follow me for decades in my teaching at various schools in the US. I'm often accused of "being fucked" for having done such research on environmental deterioration by humans leading to climate change, thus removing life.

4. Trail of Tears: Reality After A Humorous Hoax

In 1996 I was fired by the new director of the Institute of International Business in Stockholm, the one my two friends and I had started, and I had carried out the research on climate change consequences within. The firing took place at the funeral of my best friend, Gunnar Hedlund, the former director. It was then and there that I was informed by the new director that he and his Harvard associates, especially Michael Porter, had no interest in climate change stuff. I believed him.

This was similar to a prior firing I attracted in Spring, 1981 by the president of Iowa State University. That leadership fired me for a variety of reasons, but I was told by the dean that my most upsetting acts related to my teaching of climate change consequences in my architecture and engineering courses. The president spoke of his disbelief of what I taught in my design studio in the new Design Center Building. Students came to call my class "the entropy studio." The president said it was upsetting to traditional engineering professors. It was.

To demonstrate concern for climate change from business-as-usual conduct in building design and construction students became concerned and changed their attitude towards building. They removed part of a large glass wall in the classroom to the outside. It was made of stretched-skin glass and all the way around the entire building. It was to seal the building envelope. Students wanted to improve their world via low energy use cross ventilation of fresh air from nature by opening up that sealed envelope.

They replaced the section of glass skin removed with Pella double-hung windows and plywood surrounds. The Des Moines Register press was upset, as was the university president. They said it was a state-owned building and should not be touch, nor desecrated by students. The students then built a three-story house behind the design center to exaggerate their concern for their future. It was built of straw bales from soybean harvest. That was too much for Iowa State. I was thus fired, and some students were then dismissed from the School. Business as unusual was thought to be close to communism. Entropy? What the hell was that anyway?

I was then offered a job at Boston Consulting Group with part time teaching at Harvard via my 1979 dissertation. I turned that down and took a job in Newark, NJ with New Jersey Institute of Technology. I was very attracted to NJIT students. They came from poor families, had a lot of humor, and very bright minds. They had lived through the shit of life and yet continued to smile.

Due to the quality of students my NJIT projects and work turned out very well. As a Professor, an Associate Dean and then a Dean I initiated many interesting ventures that were outside the control of NJIT leadership that were locked into business as usual. Almost all my projects and works were initiated and managed by students. We did very well. When the Business School next door was about to lose its accreditation I was asked to temporarily assume its deanship role, to get it reaccredited. I began by calling for a two-day meeting of students and faculty and suspension of classes. The purpose was to map out a better future for the graduates of NJIT. The faculty were not interested and unhappy that students were allowed into such an important meeting. Thus they boycotted the second day in protest. The Chief of Staff of IBM International was running the meeting as its Chairperson and said, fine, the faculty seemed to be in way on the first day. The second day went very well. She was great.

Based on the students ideas at the meeting and their work following it the School was reaccredited at the highest possible level. It was also given the award by AACSB's President as "The Most Improved Business Program in North America." Some faculty, of course, never recovered from their deeply seated anger and were even more upset with the award given the students. It was not just my teaching of business relative to climate change that upset them. It seemed like everything I did came to upset them.

Two presidents of NJIT also came to be upset with my embracing students and their ideas for new ventures in their university, including fund raising. One president fired me as dean. He began the process ended by the second president of also firing me as a professor. The second firing took five years and five court cases. I was the first to ever have tenure removed in the history of the Institute since 1883.

Not only did NJIT Leadership dislike my teaching of climate change consequences in architecture and business classes, but my affinity for students seeming to be disrespectful to leadership? After a meeting of Institute Leadership and Faculty they concluded in a report: "If the students knew anything they would not be at NJIT taking courses." The students laughed at the comment and said: "Yup, they are right."

In 2011 the president had all files confiscated and removed from my office saying they were: "state owned property of New Jersey." This included files on my prior research, such as the 1975-77 Swedish research and its three-volume reporting, and extensive files on Exxon and other companies I worked with during the project. No files have been returned as of this time. I don't feel this is a crime against me, but certainly is against the world society that must suffer via climate change consequences in their future. Sad. Many of those files were relevant to arguments taking place in the press from 2015 to now, such as the Exxon's CEO agreeing with my research results of 1977.

In addition they seized the extensive collection of books I had in my office as used by students to supplement our discussions in class. These can be seen in the attached fifteen-page annotated bibliography. Perhaps NJIT was experimenting with an early form of confiscation of "library" books. Yes, I felt fucked, but felt students of NJIT carried a larger loss. The cost to me was trivial and predictable. Costs to students, four faculty, and an associate dean coming to my support were far greater. My costs were even more trivial in contrast to the emerging costs to life via the consequences of climate change.

5. Weaknesses, Failures, & Faults

These contents accept the earlier frustration with no progress on the climate change consequences and then move on to update our current state, where we approach and end state to life on earth, day by sad day. The following gives an outline of the last seven years via attempts to publish books as messages to those who care or are thinking of caring.

In 2018 I was contacted by an Ivy League Publisher, but not University of Pennsylvania, to reprint a book I had written in 1979 as my PhD dissertation at the Wharton School. The editor called me in 2018 saying the book had been very controversial in 1979, with the president of his university supporting its contents while others found it upsetting. His idea was it should reappear forty years after its first printing. I said fine and sent him the 1979 manuscript with an updated title. "Too Early, Too Late, Now what?" He called back to say he was unimpressed and thought it was too ambiguous for him. Would I send something clearer?

I sent him what I thus thought to be an extremely clear title: "Humans are fucked." He called to say he would never speak to me again, in his life, due to my attitude towards book publishing. I thanked him for his contribution and time. He later talked about this to others. Author House called me to say they would love to print the book that he had talked of, but with the "ambiguous" title. They did so.

A year later another publisher called to say it's time to reprint "Too Early, Too Late, Now what?" with the clear title. I said fine and sent the manuscript for "Humans are Fucked."

That humans may well be fucked is not to offend religious nor rational values. It is a metaphor of urgency for humans as they enter an increasingly hopeless and irreversible pathway.

Death provides the challenge to life's continuance. Family has long been a means to negotiate continuance within limits of the 4th dimension. Threats to life's necessary context was noted by a woman of science in 1856, Eunice Foot, a farm girl. She was concerned about a model of industrialization from fragments of analytic science. She noted the deterioration of nature from meeting bio-physical human needs and psycho-wants. CO_2 threats to conditions of life in the 3rd dimension was her concern. Now labeled climate change, it highlights consequences from man's war against nature, including diseases, chemicalized air, water, and food, then heat intolerant of life.

She illustrated how CO_2 excess could remove life from the planet. James Black of Exxon illustrated the realization of Foot's concern in 1977. He argued that humans needed alternatives to meeting bio-needs and psycho wants.

At that time David Hawk was managing an environmental deterioration research study that included Black. His final report recommended abandonment of legalistic order from analytic fragments absent any frame of context. He proposed a non-hierarchical negotiated order in a natural context without legal order governance filled with hierarchical threats shown to only encourage more deterioration.

Hawk's research emphasized creation of business as unusual. Somewhat accepted by professors in the University of Pennsylvania, it was strongly rejected by the Wharton School's Dean who argued climate change was an intellectual hoax and saw no relation between business activities and environmental deterioration. In disagreeing with the Dean students published Hawk's thesis. Much of this book comes from the 1979 student publication.

SORRY, BUT HUMANS ARE FUCKED

Climate Change from Human Limitations

HAWKEYE

They printed the book with their design of a cover as designed by their people. I liked their cover very much. The publisher did make two changes. One was adding the term "Sorry" to the beginning of my title. Two was using another name for me as author. They used my nickname that they found somewhere. It was fine. Placed in Amazon's candles, then T-shirts sections it sold well.

Humans are Fucked was a clarification of the earlier "Too Early, Too Late, Now what?" version of climate change consequences (2019). Both were updated versions of the 1979 book "Regulation of Environmental Deterioration."

> That humans may well be fucked is not to offend religious nor rational values. It is a metaphor of urgency for humans as they enter an increasingly hopeless and irreversible pathway. That path leads to death of life, or at least a fateful challenge to any of life's continuance. (From An Introduction to: *Sorry, Humans are Fucked.*)

6. Concluding Question: "Am I Really Fucked?"

The idea of having children has long been a key psychological and factual access point to human negotiations over immortality, within the limits of the 4th dimension. In this way humans can sort-of believe they control their life by controlling their death, thus via children they sort of continue on and on. It's a way to short-circuit entropy and sort of access immortality. It is consistent with the long-standing human dream to access negative entropy.

As humans walk down the stairway of life they note at about age five that attached to their neck is a death certificate. They are initially scared then become angry about that damned mortality certificate. Then they ask why death must interfere with life as promised at birth? Some note that it is natures paradox to life thus joining the contradictions of humans at war with nature. A few seek a more inquisitive, questioning of life. I hope I'm part of that second approach.

James Black was one of those special people I had the fortune to work with that rose above life's threat of death causing many to seek retaliation. Such retaliation may well explain why most humans fail to change when shown how their activities will end in elimination of much of life. As such they speak as if they are proud of working to get even with a context of nature that is essential to life's continuance. Mother nature in general and women in particular must be punished for doing such to men. Dr. Black's concern was not in that anger towards nature. He was instead concerned with an extrapolation on human behavior so that climate change would come to remove most life from our planet.

He and I had first met while I was managing an environmental deterioration research study that included the CEO of Exxon. He taught me a lot. My final report came to focus on his concern for climate change, and how it would be a consequence of environmental deterioration. He also was concerned about the thermodynamics of energy use as well as pollutants from the process. I used some of his work to argue for abandonment of a "legal order" approach from analytic fragments absent context. I then proposed a nonhierarchical negotiated order approach to reducing deterioration and climate change consequences that gave emphasis to a natural context. The regulatory method in use at the time and continuing today was based on a legal order governance as filled with hierarchical threats shown to only encourage deterioration.

Via his passion for asking why humans could be so suicidal he had no time for normal issues of promotion, pay range, and compliments from a boss. He worked as a senior scientist at Exxon. Perhaps more important was his interest in and influence by the work of a very important woman in science, Eunice Newton Foote. He used her work from 1856 to describe climate change processes then consequences to me. A later consequence would be heat intolerance of life. Black built on her illustrations of CO_2 excesses leading to removal of life from the planet to show how Foot's concern in 1856 was being realized in 1977. He argued that humans needed alternatives to coal, oil and gas in their need to meet their bio-needs and psycho wants. He later presented them to a project he was helping me with, the

Stockholm Project. In June 1977 he went on to present his ideas and my project to Exxon Chief scientists and managers in a New Jersey meeting. Foot was important to his evolution of ideas and tests.

Eunice Newton Foote was an American farm girl, and distant relative of Sir Issac Newton, who studied and taught science. Her research illustrated concern for the presumptions beneath industrialization, which were an extensive use of energy as found in the earth, to feed human desires. She showed how the process would certainly generate extensive CO_2 via expanding use of energy, such as coal, in production and product uses. She illustrated how CO_2 excess could remove life from the planet. James Black of Exxon illustrated the realization of Foot's concern in 1977. He argued that humans needed alternatives to meeting bio-needs and psycho wants. Black built on Foote's thinking and work from her speculation on how a CO_2 build-up in the atmosphere would create a climate change process. Black elaborated on this to describe a global warming process as a consequence of Exxon's products. Foote and Black had both given notice to humans on how CO_2 increase would lead to planetary life becoming deteriorated then destroyed. Blacks recommendations thus came to pose problems for Exxon's industrial future. In September of that year the Exxon CEO used Black's work to say much of what Black had said. This suggested troubles for Exxon's Board of the day.

Opposing Black's research questions was a deeply seated belief that energy discovery and use was infinitely available and essential to the human good. Expanded energy use supported expanding industrial production where the products of the process served to increased human happiness. This was consistent with prevailing management ideas regarding the overriding goal of increased productivity in creating things to meet bio-needs and psycho-wants of humans.[16] Somehow Black's research budget and the CEO's presence were removed after 1980.

A CO_2 increase would threaten conditions of life in the 3rd dimension, then aid 4th dimensional entropic elimination of it. Entropic processes were just being clarified in 1856 but she seemed

---

[16] David Hawk, Sorry, Humans are Fucked,

to have a sense of thermodynamic rules. Death is a hindrance to life's continuance. As mentioned, family has long been the means to negotiate continuance within limits of the 4th dimension. Having children has long been the path to immortality. The second major avenue to humans threatening to remain immortal is religion, and the warfare essential to it.

Climate change now threatens life. The science of it highlights consequences from man's war against nature, including diseases, chemicalized air, water, and food, then heat intolerance of life. Human activities came to create removal of life in the 4th dimension at an accelerated rate. Labeled climate change, it highlighted consequences from man's question to fill psycho-wants while destroying anything that gets in the way.

II

LEARNING FROM DEMISE: A MAYAN CIVILIZATION

1. What Went Wrong in Yucatan?

Even though my story was not new in the history of life, many felt I had been uniquely fucked, over and over. Some even believed there was no PhD resulting from my concern about something so questionable as climate change. Their comments mostly came from the time and trouble I had faced in gaining approval to study such a subject. Much of this was settled twenty years later in a European Conference on environmental concerns as they were growing in the world, not just in the nations in Hawk's early study. Many had begun to see that the study of environmental deterioration and its management was a worthwhile area of concern, yet they thought any answers were in the technological and the regulatory, both areas that I had shown to be questionable as posing solutions to climate change consequences.

I introduced a study I did in 1969 of the fall of the Mayan Civilization. I studied there for a semester. In 1989 such a study was more acceptable and began to be seen relative to my climate change concern in 1979. By 2019 the comparison of what happened to Mayan cities and is happening to World cities is amazingly similar.

There of course continues to be much disagreement about the nature of the world in 1975, as well as 1875 but to introduce responses I clarify such by asking: Which scientist, from which discipline, will write the most significant book ever written by a human? The title will be something like: *"On the End of Species."* Such a book will be the memorable obituary of humankind on a bookshelf. At the other end of the shelf will be the book giving its support to human pursuance of industrial development in 1859. That book was titled: "On the Origin of Species." In between can be a nice collection of literature presenting the depth allowed in human optimism with the dreams of reason as realized via industrialization. These can cover the expansion of the human spirit from the technological as supported by a version of the scientific, while dreaming of an artificially intelligent future. The process avoids looking into the decline of various civilizations.

We show a misguided faith in what might best be called humanism. Armed with arrogance and steeped in ignorance we created a 150-year history of optimism about being human, but which ended up with a history of the demise of the human condition based on what humans did. We seem to be similar in our behavior to the Mayan's thus we will see the demise of humans and all forms of life in the human context. This is easy to see across the planet in 2020, not restricted to Yucatan. Being trapped in the results of cause-effect analysis only obscures our seeing this.

We seem to be on a suicidal trek, called progress. Our measures of such stem from an ever increasing measure of productively doing the wrong things, in the wrong way. I say such harsh things as I am mostly trying to communicate with myself. If you can gain anything from the echoes of my sentences to me I will be less sad.

Perhaps it helps us understand, as such did for the group in attendance to the conference mentioned before, to see aspects of what is moving towards our civilization by looking to prior civilizations. Herein I offer the Mayan as an example. that essentially disappeared via climate changing to its context. In existence for almost 2,500 years it did well. Our industrial-based and driven civilization has developed in only 200 years and is disabling much of the globe, not just the province of Yucatan.

2. A Societal Collapse, Not The End State of Life

The Mayan Civilization began around 1500 B.C.E. and ended about 900 C.E. It's demise began then reached a low point between 850 and 1000. Its greatest achievements occurred from 250 C.E. until 900 C.E. Now seen as a very sophisticated collection of humans they understood scientific principles. Such let them to major inventions such as a means to regulate forty cities without central control, development of a sophisticated currency and trade systems to unite the cities. During their most robust period they had five to ten million citizens occupying more than 40 cities.

They are perhaps best known for a remarkable access to astronomical understanding. They developed unique methods for tracking the movements of the sun, moon, and various planets. Their civilization mostly disappeared in the 16th century via the arrival of the Spanish invaders and becoming subjected to their demands and culture. They build an infrastructure of inlaid stone roads to connect their cities and the larger world. Archeologists were long mystified by how they could have created such a network of cities with sophisticated roadways yet did not seem to know of the wheel. In 1969 they were excavating a cenote and what they found changed everything, reducing the former knowledge base to mostly question marks. A child's toy was discovered with wheels on it; thus they certainly knew of the wheel but perhaps didn't make much utilitarian use of it as their major god was the circle.

In January 1969 I returned to Iowa State University, college of engineering and architecture, to complete my studies. In 1966 I had been drafted out of the university and sent to Vietnam for two years. I didn't much care for being on the campus and found that as a student I could organize and take a study trip to another country, and the university would pay for my hiring of instructors, as long as I opened the study trip up to other students. I thus decided to go visit Merida, Yucatan to study architecture of that region while also studying the archeology of Ancient Maya peoples. Our key design studio would focus on design of a naval new town for the Minister of Navy.

The New Town idea by the Navy was cancelled so I then contacted the famous Dr. Victor Segovia Pinto, an archeologist. I asked for his recommendation for what to study in Yucatan. He offered to come help teach the class coming to visit the university in Merida for a semester and visiting the abandoned ancient Mayan cities. He eagerly agreed to help us and recommended our using the ancient city of Chichin-Itza, near Merida as a base.

We thus learned much about an extensive attempt at creating a civilization that came to fail via climate changes to its region. The society of Chichen-Itza had worked hard and gone far to develop ever more sophisticated agriculture to feed the millions housed in the neighboring sophisticated cities. They came to remove many trees an wilderness of nature in an expansion of development to meet human needs, and wants.

3. Ignorance of Experts, As Revealed by a Toy

Work at Chichen-Itza came to change the assumptions for understanding of Mayan civilization, technology, and necessary infrastructures. Early on we were told via research documents on anthropology at the US National Museum that the Mayan's had not discovered the leading European technology of the day, e.g., wheels. Authors of that idea expanded to suggested that the Mayans would have been a highly developed civilization had they known of the wheel.

During the 1960s a child's toy, depicted below, was discovered. Scholars were amazed that it had wheels on it. This brought into question much else that was known about Mayan development. Later scientists have argued that sure, since the wheel was the shape of their Sun God, they avoided using it on vehicles. If course, this did not solve the foremost question of what was used on the very elaborate roadways between cities built of implanted stones. god. What was the alternative to the use of wheels? Students in my group loved the dilemma.

Towards 800 AD the region began to see a drought which closed much of the agriculture thus closing many of the cities. Only the small villages continued as they were closest to what food was left in the society. It proved to be a fascinating study abroad mission for the ISU students. Twenty-two additional students joined my venture. We never recovered from what we had learned about humans, change, weather, governments, and culture.

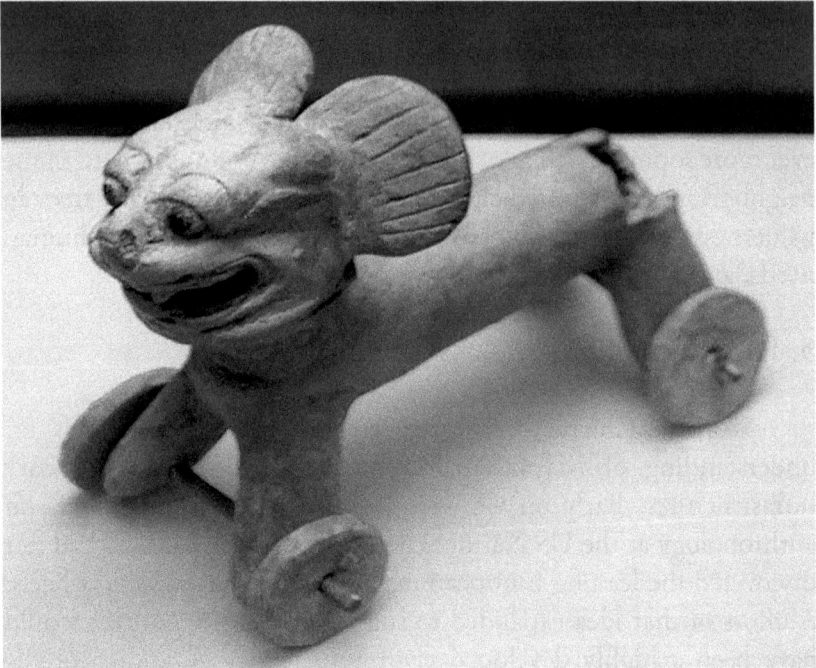

The Child's Toy with "Wheels," found during our visits.

A good friend, and supporter of me as a difficult student, Prof. Karl Kochimski, provided cover for my organizing such a trip, as it was against university leadership.

Somehow the Maya's were attractive to me as they had come to be fucked by changes in their context, presumably an early version of climate change and its consequences. They had some responsibility for what went wrong. In the providing of additional farmland for the expanding society many trees and wildlife were removed. This was an emphasis during 100 years of late-stage development. Then, a drought emerged then took over the region that for so long had supported bountiful food production.

What does this now say to inform us of the world of 2024 where it also sees a context being changed by human ideas, and actions. We too begin to see instabilities that follow erratic weather changes that provide too little and too much water. Best guesses believe the lack of food production resulting from the known drought led to civil wars coupled to a decline in those well-known and prosperous trade relations in Mesoamerica. The prior stability provided by predictable and dependable rain never returned.

The class has trouble conceptualizing the situation and its end state. Our Spanish teaching at the university noticed this and the unhappiness that resulted. She advised us to stop seeking the causes of such effects, as there were many and most will never be known. I recalled her when I began in 1975 to think about effects arising from prior systemic effects, not particular causes that were not.

4. Where Were They? Where Are We?

(ACCEPTING OUR BEING FUCKED MAY BE A KEY TO BECOMING UN-FUCKED)

It's helpful to look backward to prior catastrophes in human civilizations as they give clues of how bad things can become without much warning or explanation to those involved. As the Mayan grew and expanded their success into 40 cities with millions of residents, then turned more of nature into agriculture to feed those people change had been initiated. Relative to what we see as approaching climate change consequences the Mayan use of Yucatan was quite small in contrast to the conditions of the world going through similar human induced changes. Important for us is the impact not the scale. It can happen again to humans.

The impending fate of life on the planet is becoming seen as an effect of climate change consequences. Herein the concept of consequences is key. It will be used to describe the effects of prior effects.

Formerly called second order results of results, consequences were generally unnoticed. Where noted they became purposefully ignored and not seen as prior effects floating disconnected to the effects that were underway.

As was suggested before we long used cause-effect connections to develop knowledge and pose predictions. That was quite limited and can now be seen as contributing to this process we call climate change. Cause-effect logic of humans gave us lots of disassembled parts into parts where the ultimate part could be patented as reward for the thinker. Using the relations between the parts and the consequences of their effects was avoided. As will be described in greater detail that approach left to us by our Greek fathers no longer provides sense nor allows access to sense. Climate change consequences void such limits of unaided rationality as well as the logic on which it was based.

- *Logic*, n. The art of thinking and reasoning in strict accordance with the limitations and incapacities of the human misunderstanding. The basic of logic is the syllogism, consisting of a major and minor premise and a conclusion – thus:
- *Major Premise*: Sixty men can do a piece of work sixty times as quickly as one man.
- *Minor Premise*: One man can dig a post hole in sixty seconds: therefore, a rational conclusion:
- Sixty men can dig a posthole in one second.
- This may be called the syllogism arithmetical, in which by combining logic and mathematics, we obtain a double certain and are twice blessed.[17]

In 2024 we might say anyone relying on existing logic to help manage cause-effect thinking is fucked. Likewise, anyone thinking going deeper into cause-effect logic to find a way to manage climate

---

[17] Ambrose Bierce, *The Devil's Dictionary*, New York: American Century Series, 1957, P. 109. (Written 1881)

change consequences is also fucked. This is not intended as an insult in that much of my live has been organized around the misfortunes of being fucked. Perhaps the following will help introduce you to the meaning of such.

5. History of Human Hawk

I have seen little change in human thinking about their being predominant over all other things since working in the family garden on the farm when I was four. I could not understand why humans needed to be so artificial and in opposition to the natural. Back then, I remember asking why is it this way? My family thought I was funny. I thought their use of straight rows of only one plant species was funny.

1. At thirteen I was banned from attendance in my local church for related questions.
2. At fifteen I was elected president of my 4H chapter. My first act was to close it as many members treated their animals badly and should not hide that problem in the shadow of 4H.
3. At seventeen I became president of my local Future Farmers of America Chapter. I had campaigned to halt a high school program set up to make the world an obviously better place. The program assigned points to students who brought in bags of animal and bird parts, including heads, to school on Monday mornings. School employees would then inspect and assign points. This had been set up to extinguish the local pests and varmints. Such was thought to support a better life. The Monday morning inspections revealed much. Shocking to some, but not me, was how the occasional cat or dog came to be defined as a pest. I managed to get the Administration to suspend the program to research its consequences, but only for a bit. Via anger school leadership got even with me. They banned

me from taking any college preparatory courses during the remainder of my high school attendance.

4. At eighteen I was given the Isaac Walton award for the above and also for writing an article in the local newspaper that kept local government from removing a large bird-filled tree from a stream. Government officials had argued how modern life would be improved and made safer for humans if storm waters could ran away faster. The tree was saved from local governance.

5. At twenty-eight I had responsibility for an Environmental Impact Statement Review. It was for a proposed ten-thou-sand-person housing development in Florida. After the review process it gained Federal and State approval. I had recommended a design which proposed the retention of swamps and minimal human impacts to the site's nature. I then presented the approval document to the developer. He threw it and the proposed design into his trash can say-ing: "Now we can get to work." He preferred business as usual, the clearing and leveling of the property.

6. At thirty I entered the Wharton School PhD program in systems sciences. The research described herein was carried out and written up while in that program. It was a sci-ence program, but I avoided science steeped in cause-effect charting from analytical thinking after segmenting, reduc-ing and redacting problems.

7. My work continues to be consistent with systems sciences. It looks at problems in terms of relationships, always in a context, and avoids seeing effects abstracted from causes so causes can be regulated, governed, or managed absent their meaningful context.

Regardless of the widespread selling of optimism I have seen lit-tle change in human values, those connections of thinking to behav-ing, since I was four. Perhaps there is now greater anger, but it seems to be mostly directed at disappointment in our not getting what we thought was promised to us by life, including from the environment and from others. The research discussed herein represents a major departure from usual research into bits of optimism floating in a mess of humanism. As was said someplace before: "Humans Are Fucked."

After the concern for environmental deterioration seen herein was presented to faculty of the Wharton School, it was found acceptable a year later by seven professors at the University. Five ended up being drawn from schools outside of business. They focused on seven questions during their review. The questions reveal much about the review process, more than the research topic, and its context.

a) *Why would a student in the Wharton Business School attempt research into the prognosis of human continuance relative to growing environmental deterioration from economic activities?* I responded at the time that it appeared as a good doorway into problems in business and humans that mattered.

b) *Why would business school faculty advisors allow such?* My advisors — Russell Ackoff, Hasan Ozbekhan, and Eric Trist – strongly supported what I believed I should work on. All three were unusual humans. Based on their stature in the university the concern against my work was dropped.

c) *Why did the research need to be moved to Sweden, and not be based in the USA?* I asked the committee to reference any similar research projects they could find based in US institutions. They found none on the subject as framed, with such enthusiastic governmental and corporate involvement, especially not at US business schools.

d) *Why did the three-member review committee of 1978 need to be expanded to five, with two from engineering departments, then expanded again with two more from science departments?* The project was seeking more than causes of effects thus a more systemic representation group was required.

e) *Why did it take more than one year of committee review to gain approval of the evidence in the thesis?* Normal review is a few weeks. The notes from their meetings showed committee members' concern with ideas about humans as a cause of future tragedy via environmental consequences. In addition, some were concerned about speculating on ideas like climate change coming to the planet. They wanted it dropped. It was kept.

f) *Why did Wharton's Dean refuse to sign off on the approved document?* He commented: "I do not see what environmental deterioration has to do with business." I responded to him agreeing with his statement. He clearly did not see the connection.

Only one of the four approved volumes made it to the University of Pennsylvania Library archives. Then, why was that one not forwarded to dissertation documents arrive at University of Michigan under global PhD Abstracts? As a footnote on the above process seemingly willed by a number of decision-makers in university systems, how did NJIT come to join the filtration process? My professor's office at NJIT was filled with many books, papers, documents, and past research reports on climate change. My classes seemed to appreciate them as their library for going deeper into a number of research interests. The book portion is listed in the attached appendix. Could it have any relationship to the mind of the past Director of the Honors Center of NJIT who repeatedly asked the dean overseeing my courses to remove me from teaching honor's students? He held a doctorate in education but no past in the sciences. He found climate change issues upsetting and possibly also thought they were a hoax. He was especially upset by my teaching of business as unusual. In 2011 he and the then president of NJIT had my office contents confiscated. Included were my last copies of the three research conclusion volumes and a copy of the original dissertation. It has never been returned to me despite requests. I was told by an Associate Dean that the past president had them burned. As commented earlier, there were thirteen boxes removed from my office with six of them containing my books. We now label them as: "missing in inaction." Past students label this as "business as usual" in universities.

III

IMPEDIMENTS TO LIFE: MASCULINE LOGIC OF CAUSE-EFFECT

The sad humor behind all this can be seen in how humans work to mask the key behaviors from the past leading to an extinct future. We will examine this limitation of a human way of knowing: creating knowledge via discovering the causes of effects.

1. Cause-Effect Thinking, An Unfortunate History

Cause-effect logic has long been a doorway into a world where seeing context has been placed by seeking reduction of reality into pieces of pieces of pieces, etc. You know what I mean if you paid attention to the process of a normal education. Herein I will argue to upgrade this death spiral for the mind and instead include more a context as an actor. I will argue for experimenting with thinking of the effects of the past creating the effects of the future. It's like a divorce court where a judge seeks the cause of the dissolution of the relationship. Is it the yelling, beating, lying or purchase of a gun? This logic leads to much of what humans do to solve their problems and helps explain why the problem thus worsens instead of finding resolution. This is how we walked backward into the solution of recycling even though it was and is shown to be negative entropy in character.

Instead of these funny tangents from a context of hate it is the predictable effect of becoming formally married to freeze the formerly fluid relationship thus removing the natural humor. The couple then resorts to individualized concentration on themselves, their cars, psycho-wants, and related human excursions into the strange. Retention of means to apply fluid management in a fluid, i.e., alive, would be more natural. Lacking a deep connection to life, and the living, we get in our cars and approach extinction in a manner that ensures its sooner than later. No, I do not consider myself an "environmentalist" and have never been called such. To me such is a person that bought their summer home last year.

Now we need to understand the alternative to local cause-effect thinking so we might better understand the phenomena that emerge from climate change consequences. Hereafter they will be noted in a short form of C-Cubed, or C^3. When we rely on cause-effect analysis to understand such we generally end in a truly disjointed analysis of what in fact never was. Doing such mostly creates one of the favorite pastimes of human thought, creating complexity that buries identity as well as its soul in the Faustian sense of bargaining over the short-term gains to avoid the long-term pains of that which we mostly do.

The more intelligent seem to not know what to do about it, or continuance of life on their planet. Less intelligent, who use the noises from their openings to sit back and watch storms expand via manful comments about climate having always changed. The rest of us reflect on our teachings from parents, associates, churches, and schools to compare what was said with what is being occupied. The only truth seems to be that our knowledge base is increasingly irrelevant to continuance of life as contrast with the news of drought, flood, storms, and inflation is cost of what is essential to life, not that which reduces the value of neighbors. Thus, some of us argue how we must act immediately to correct things, yet don't know how to act, what would be correct, or even what needs to be corrected. Our image is of being frozen in front of 2-D AI computer, phone, TV, etc. images while reality moved into 4-D seeking 5-D. Poor humans. Can we change?

> "It's not working, and we are unsure how to define work, or it."[18]

The manner in which we live ensures a bad end and no chance for the life of grandchildren. Thus, we pursue our sad end with little enthusiasm. Meanwhile, those with resources to have cars drive around asking what is climate change stuff? It seems serious so what is the solution to this threat to individualized mortality tomorrow to mass erasure today? Surely our leadership knows more than we? Maybe we should pull over at the next exit from this highway to hell, find a beautiful tree to relax under while we consider a re-definition of human beings, being human. Didn't life face five previous episodes with extinction from the planet? Didn't humans face periods of needing to seriously redefine the human experience such as a falling Rome, a Medieval reorientation, and a post WWII attempt at managing the downside of human behavior? Clearly, we need to seek a more complementary meaning to life. Its current definition shifting back and forth between the Garden of Eden and Darwin is beginning to be seen as extraordinarily dangerous, even suicidal. A small but growing number of scientists are staring into the cosmos asking the once banned question: "Are we fucked?"[19]

It's interesting to note the parallel avenues being travelled by pro-creators of climate change and the anti-abortionists. The major-

---

[18] The closing sentence in a farewell lecture to students at New Jersey Institute of Technology. They asked me to give such after being fired by Robert Altenkirch and Chris Christie, and before I was banned from campus. 8 charges were brought then dismissed due to no evidence. 25 charges were then created with a judge finding me guilting of one charge, based on him not being able to detect changes or erasures on a xerox of a report. Spring, 2008. Newark, NJ. Lecture titled: "The Importance of It's Too Late."

[19] Amy Sohn, *The Man Who Hated Women*, New York: Farrar, Straus and Giroux, 2021.

ity of both groups are men and rely on cause-effect examples to justify their wrong views.

This book concentrates on the climate change roadway and its consequences but it seems helpful to keep the abortion issue in the discussion as it clarifies the thinking of the masculine mind. This is seen in some important historic comments of one-hundred and fifty years ago.

2. 1873 Comstock Act: Manly Management of It All

Much of this section comes from the work of Sara Chase in the 1870's. She made many public postings and thus became a central target of a masculine enterprise to keep women in their place. There was uncertainty as to how to define that place except it must be below men. Sara Chase made many postings in journals about men like the infamous Comstock, who "fathered" a Congressional law against female speech, concerns for their body, nature, and well-being of life. For purposes herein the Comstock venture represented the majority of highly placed men who wanted the lower classes to remain low via giving them orders, with a focus on legal orders. An important type of order was against obscenity with the work "fuck" at central stage.

> "Comstock did not understand 'the difference between obscenity and science.' Everything which pertains to the organs of reproduction, whether presented with a view to instruction in regard to their physiology and hygiene, or to inflame the lewd passions of the lower nature, all to his mind are alike vile, and he forthwith proceeds to exercise the power vested in him, in conformity to his perverted judgment."[20]

None-the-less Comstock managed to get the "Comstock Act signed into law on Monday, March 3, 1873, as he became 29 years of age. He was a store clerk in a clothing store, not a member of

---

[20] Ibid., p. 143.

Congress but Congressional members followed his ideas closely in drawing up the Comstock Act. "His law" was then amended three months later to firm up its enforcement. Thus, any possession of obscene matter would be punished by two years of hard labor and a $5,000 fine. Included in obscenity was any act to attempt control of abortion. The Act has yet to be rescinded. Few Americans, especially few men, now seem ready to have an open discussion on why a woman's mid-section inherently belongs to men, for their "caretaking."

The downside of this model is deep and widely distributed to where it is not needed nor wanted. This can be seen with clarity in examples related to the theme of this book. One hundred and fifty years ago the United States Government addressed the fucked issue as raised herein along with the eternal masculine fight to keep the feminine in servitude via a law manifesting changelessness to protect society from the challenges of change. In March 1873 Congress passed the Comstock Act, still mostly in effect today and clarified by the US Supreme Court recently in disallowing women to own themselves via owning their bodies.

That act prohibited dissemination of any "…article of an immoral nature, of any drug or medicine, of any article whatever for the prevention of contraception or precuring of abortion" through the U.S. mail of across state lines. That law forbids placing "fucked" in print. Probably the law, still on the books, should be seen as "women are fucked" as the writer of it, Anthony Comstock, a store clerk Congregationalist from New York City, illustrated extreme hatred for women.

He defined women as "the obscene." Even more obscene was his anti-feminine law whose constitutionality was upheld three times (1957, 1971, and 1977) via a rational that the First Amendment to the US Constitution does not "protect obscene speech." Opposition to the act came from individuals like Margaret Sanger, who was reported to stand as a "radical," fighting for taking back the rights of women as stolen by some men. Her issues included the female right to birth control. She put instructions on this out via her monthly newspaper. She described birth control methods and attracted Emma Goldman to side with her in giving lectures on Sanger.

Their past discussions continue to be referenced. Most recently they were in discussions in 2023 cases on drugs used to stop or prevent pregnancy. The masculine will be seriously criticized herein as mostly responsible for the wrong in human conduct and most recently behind propagating a form of industrialization.

The laws passed in several states in the past few years move towards firming up the Comstock Act while treating climate change concerns as a scientific hoax. Thus we can see how similar values, mostly of the masculine, seem to surround the ideas of climate change consequences returning to humans from how they live, as well as reaffirmation of the Garden of Eden story about the value(s) of women. Some studies say 70% of humans believe very harsh consequences are waiting in the future from human acts ending in climate change from the past. Other studies say that percentage only relates to scientists who study climate change consequences. The majority of humans continue undeterred on their well-traveled speedway to the end. They are fine with continuance of business as usual, especially when they are confused.

Based on all known climate change consequences arriving sooner than initially expected there is some certainty that in twenty-five years we will be trying to make sense of life via new definitions of what and who we are. Some will of course be quite angry about their early 20th Century movie story lines having silly endings questioned. They may even have access to nuclear tools with which they can teach others a lesson about what is and isn't.

Thus with the Comstock Act and all the similar Acts from an American Congress we see a guarantee of species suicide that carries us into furtherance of climate change consequences. Such Acts and the emphasis on the paper on which they are written continues the two-dimensional framework of humans now found in books, cinema, TVs, computers, and mobile phones.

This Comstock Act can best be understood as a modern replay of what kept those living in Plato's Cave duly locked in place. They sat there with heads in a framework forcing them to stare at the two dimensions of information placed on a shadowed ceiling from shadows generated by an energy fed campfire.

3. The Masculine War Against The Natural

To understand this, we need to clarify ideas about being human, being alive, being in a context, and seeing a divergence between cosmic and human nature. As a minimum we need to see the contradictions resulting from such. For example, we know entropy to be a sacrosanct law of the universe as we watch human attempt to live outside such restrictions via negative entropy ideals. Upon reflection we see the cost of such in negative consequential expansion of entropy effects. For example, to avoid reflecting on the entropic consequences of a kitchen we badly designed and roughly built we leave and go for a drive in our care to pretend it didn't and doesn't matter. To begin to redesign the process we can begin rethinking a science based on the limitations of cause-effect conceptualization. As it's simple-minded we can continue to use such in parlor games, as long as we pretend the open system is beyond the closed doors. That was how IT, cybernetics, systems analysis, breeding, etc. came to represent negative entropy in life.

Humans have long reflected on their own nature as from a hierarchical being that deemed them to cause improvements in life's understanding and evolution. This could come from a God, a philosopher-king like Plato or a Cambridge educated man seeing all life evolving via a central source such as Darwin. All such hierarchical thinking places nature in the position of a stage-set, or backdrop to what matters. Meanwhile humans can thus reform their thinking of themselves at the center of life in the universe, perhaps even the central reason for its existence. This is seen in thousands of years of the history of humans. For raising questions about this idea of manifest destiny in humans Socrates was sent to death by his societal context, and Plato's enlightened escapees from his cave to tell them of a very enlightened world out in the light brought them to a similar fate. Students today that raise questions, not memorizing answers, become similarly burdened in life.

Humans seem fixated on the belief that they are, even must be, at the center of the universe, solar system, earth, corporation, or social group they occupy. They shun the mind of the inquisitive and embrace the ongoing inquisitions of humankind in continual searches for the disobedient amongst them. Somehow humans find the egocentric to be trustworthy when difficulties approach the group. This is how they define a natural order that suits their values. As such context is defined as resources for feeding of the egocentric. The values of the natural and the larger role thus played in forming and reforming context become lost. This is known as the religion of human life as depicted in the book, the Arrogance of Humanism, that describes how humans use context as raw materials that end in empires of dirt. In the end this becomes destructive of context.

Evidence that earth and its occupants are not at the center of anything grow, even though the consequences of avoiding such knowledge still grow. In the following there are four quotes by two serious thinkers about the human role in it all. It begins in the science of Stephen Hawking and ending in poetry of Leonard Cohen.

> "The human race is just a chemical scum on a moderate-sized planet, orbiting around a very average star in the outer suburb of one among a hundred billion galaxies. We are so insignificant that I can't believe the whole universe exists for our benefit. That would be like saying that you would disappear if I closed my eyes."[21]

A situational awareness suggesting a desperate need to change is beginning to emerge at the edge of what we call human nature. This appears to come from signs of trouble in our context along with ideas of a greater good awaiting human participation. The options for responding to the looming bad, a bad that threatens the context that defines and supports life as we know it, are fading. There may well be great potential for accessing the greater good in life if humans find ways to participate in it in a different manner. The evidence for historic definitions of human egocentricities and how they destroy context is growing. Something seems clearly wrong in business as usual.

---

[21] Stephen Hawking, From an interview with Ken Campbell on Reality on the Rocks: Beyond Our Ken, 1995.

Humans seem to be going out of business. It becomes clearer with time that humans must change, or nature will change their definition of existence. They will fail to remain as part of life in the universe.

> "I think computer viruses should count as life...I think it says something about human nature that the only form of life we have created so far is purely destructive. We've created life in our own image." [22]

Change of humans seems essential to survival but does that mean anything relative to the human definition of progress that they have followed for at least the past two thousand years. That was the search for the mechanical, then the mechanical organized into the industrial. Therein productivity of operations became more valued than evaluation of the product and consequences of its use. Its as if Adam Smith was the Godhead of thinking long before he lived. Change in this is urgently needed, as the theme of making mistakes ever more efficiently is the rule of business, not experiments in less efficiency in finding the right. Russell Ackoff long preached this idea to corporations he advised. Sometimes it mattered.

We know activities that denigrate then deteriorate the environments we depend upon are in growing need of increasingly urgent change. Seeing drought-controlled field non-growth next to storm-destroyed barns informs us of much if we take note. How then do we control our conscious management of those acts that lead to such counter-productive results? How do we access our unconscious, that storehouse of beliefs that define values for what to do and not do?

We used to pray to someone's gods or negotiate with self-designed devils in dealing with questions such as those above. When natural intelligence reorganizes our thinking we soon will see how those early gods and devils were simply earlier versions of the now looming promises of artificial intelligence. Will AI help improve our relations to our more essential natural intelligence and the nature it

---

[22] Stephen Hawking, from a speech at Macworld Expo, Boston, 1994.

represents? Just now it seems that something more, and/or less, will be required. As nature becomes more endangered and thus protective against its human enemy we shall see. Herein hope is not with the promises of AI. Those offered by the early proponents of AI, and its digital basis, Parmenides, Plato, and Aristotle, did not seem to improve the human role in setting conditions of life.

> "Ring the bells that still can ring, forget your perfect offering, there is a *crack*, a *crack* in everything that's how the *light gets in...*"[23]

A call to change generally attracts youthful spirits and elderly feelings awaken from decades of life failures encircling them. As a member of the second group, I struggle with the history seen in the variety and veracity of humanly inspired wrongs. Most of these wrongs arise from large celebrations of homocentricity as the basis of the universe, before they are shown to be trivial. Those with an ability to reflect wonder from where this all comes and to where it all will go. They watch other humans continually engage in arguments, much drama, and even more anger. The trivial nature of the results gets hidden by our self-creation of complexity out there when our often-used expression "it's complicated" fails to have meaning. To avoid all this I reduce the struggle with humans and what they don't know to: "It's the fight against shit, that's what it's all about." Clarification of "it" then shows how the more real relates to what changes, not the less real attempt to create changelessness. Via accepting change as natural we come to appreciate the "it" before "it's too late."

A danger in your battles with shit is that you tend to get some on you that is difficult to remove. This explains why lawyers and police in societies are thought to operate at a lower standard than those they attempt to regulate. On a more personal level we see this in reflecting on the cost to us in pointing out the bad, to find a greater good, we usually seem to wait, thinking the greater good can come later. Except in our dreams that greater good is seldom found.

---

[23] Leonard Cohen, from the album *The Future*, the song "Anthem," 1992.

Such is seen in Goethe's Faustian play, part I and especially in part II. I will not go into the Faustian take on being human where the human sells his soul to the devil in youth to have wealth, intelligence, and a beautiful woman beside him in life but no greater good via a soul at the end. This is a European depiction of the problem of being human. Paul Valery's version of the Faustian Tragedy at the end of WWII is more appropriate to America. The devil he depicts is fearful of negotiating with Americans and is in hiding from them. They are a bit crazy, with their souls easily available to any buyer at little to no cost.

This human situation will herein be described differently. It is the embracing of the selling of negative entropy in the short-term in hopes to finding resources to manage real entropy in eternal-time. We see this in business school courses where we learn to market products as needing no energy nor maintenance during their life. This is to build our wealth so we may come to create better products using less energy and reduced service, as if Ayn Rand were directing the operation. A better definition of humans and their role in the life of the universe may be the opposite of the Ayn Rand type, more akin to the inspiration of Joan of Arc.

As Mark Twain concluded from his study of her life:

> She is easily and by far the most extraordinary person the human race has ever produced. ....It took six thousand years to produce her; her likeness will not be seen in the earth again in fifty thousand.[24]

4. Human Beings: Fucked By The Masculine

From age seven on I was expected to work as a farmer on the farms of my father. That was why I was born and tolerated by fathers, or so neighboring fathers would tell me. As I dealt with no other children except my brother I assumed this was the way things needed to be.

---

[24] Mark Twain, *Person Recollections of Joan of Arc*, 1896.

I was told to milk twenty-some cows each morning and evening at 5 o'clock thus there was no time or reason for socializing with others over life and its meaning. During hay baling times I was expected to ride on the hay bailer to clip the two ends of the wire ties together even though the dust from the hay plunger was to often so thick I could see nothing, and others thought I was a bale of hay at the end of each day's work. One day a neighbor boy invited me to join him swimming in a local creek. Knowing the life I was living was pretty bad I went with him for four hours during the heat of the day and disregarded my need to be on the hay baler. When I got home my father asked if it was worth it, then beat me with a rubber hose sufficiently that I could not sit on what was beaten. I learned many things that day, none of them good, nor giving access to the optimistic. I thought humans were fucked.

When I was eighteen, I was told by my uncle that if I was thinking of going to college, I shouldn't go to Iowa State University. It's too hard. Per subject I should avoid electrical engineering. It's hard. As I did not think much of his life nor his advice I of course when to Iowa State University and studied Electrical Engineering. My father was in the front yard shaking his fist at me when I left for college. I found ways to work nights to pay for housing, food and tuition as no funding was available. When I got to the university I met a black student that I quickly liked. We became best friends, and both joined the Air Force ROTC to get a bit of pay and socialize.

The next Spring there was a special day to learn about respect for authority and taking orders. We were forced to carry a cigars box of candy treats around our necks as we walked around campus in our uniforms. Upper class ROTC members were to stop us and sift through our boxes to find candy or treats they liked, as they order us to respect them and do push-ups, etc. My friend and I noted that they really liked chicklet gum tablets as they could cram an entire box in their mouths while yelling at us. For an entire day we tolerated what seemed like an unusually disgusting exercise. That night we noted that Feen-A-Mint Oral tablets, for constipation, looked much like Chicklet tablets. Thus we decided to help those humans that seemed rather dumb and ugly by replacing the Chicklets with Feen-A-Mint tablets. We watched the upper classmen behave the same the next day. That night a special assembly was called for the ISU auditorium, where we were told of all the stomach sickness on campus of ROTC men and we two were formally ejected from ROTC. We were told we were fucked and needed to change. The behavior of those harassing us was applauded for helping the great good of society.

Two years later I transferred into architecture upon listening to one of worst people I ever saw giving a lecture on the future of architecture in controlling humans through greater use of roughly exposed concrete surfaces. I felt I needed to do battle with such a human, so I transferred my major. My local draft board then sent me a letter condemning me for what I had done. They pointed out that I had transferred from a four-year program to a five-year program, but they would draft me at the end of four, as I just have changed to avoid being drafted one additional year. I sent them back a letter saying they should take me immediately if that was their attitude, and besides "fuck you." I did such for humor as I knew by law they could not draft me then. None-the-less, they did draft me the next week.

"Fuck-you" can prove to be expensive.

1) Saying FU to my draft board, thus ending up in Vietnam for seventeen months.
2) Being charged with insubordination under battle conditions.
3) Being given the Outstanding Professor Award by Alumni of NJIT
4) Asked to not use FU when talking of how awards were issued.
5) Fired for suggesting the University President needed sports due to his maybe having a small penis.

From these episodes with others I came to place a sign in my university office saying: "It's The Fight Against Shit, That's What It's All About." This was to depict that "Humans Were at War with Nature," which in fact was with their own nature, then the nature of others, and finally with all of nature. Then we arrive at the question of why is war so important to humans, especially to the masculine?

The challenges of one's life are especially clear during war time. For me it was a war in Vietnam. It was a war of the ugly and the dumb. I watched how leadership was or became mostly leadershit. Signs of continuance of such continue today. During Vietnam leaders would order the dumb to find horrible ways for the wrong to kill the wrong, with horrible consequences in the vulnerability of the innocent. Women and children came to pay the costs, especially while fleeing from men. During all this, the love of my life, a beautiful Vietnamese woman in Danang, came to be killed as the cost for knowing me.

During a Tet Offense at Khe Sanh, in late January 1968, I was ordered to shoot at fleeing women and children. I suggested to the captain that I would feel better if I simply shoot him. For some reason he took it badly. During a hearing under battle conditions, I explained my disrespect. This comment came to be repeated by many for many years: "We the unwilling, led by the unqualified, to kill the unfortunate, die for the ungrateful." I was recommended for promotion.

Forty years later I was again challenged by a president of a school called NJIT for "insubordination" to lawful authority. Located in Newark, NJ, I was a temporary dean after being asked to keep the university trustees from closing the school due to bad performance. During two years, via allowing those who had the most to lose from being at a bad school, the students, to lead the school, became highly regarded in the region and nation. During a two-day suspension of classes, a meeting was held of all those interested in the school's future, where the students led the meeting, and faculty avoided attending the second day. The Chief of Staff for IBM served as the Chairperson of the meeting. During the second day we discovering a basis for a new mission and thus a highly advanced school of learning.

When the president received the reaccreditation notice, saying we had the most improved business school in North America that year, he fired me. He said it was for ignoring his dream of NCAA membership as the route to success. I had commented that those needing exaggerated sports in a science and technology university might be motivated from too small genitalia. (I made a similar comment to Donald Trump in 1994, in Atlantic City, relative to a proj-

45

ect I was doing on a regulation free zone in a city. He asked to be involved in the project. I thus closed it.)

NJIT leadership organized meetings, hearings and trials around trivial laws interpreted for their self-interests. It took five years, not the hour required during a battle in Vietnam. In the New Jersey situation there were five court cases over five years, where all were lost. The judge managing the process was paid $500/hour by the university to ensure his respect for authority and I came to like him even if he found me guilty of one of 25 charges the president had posed as criminal. We had not progressed very far from the Khe Sanh battlefield idea of leadership in forty years. It was not the fault of those involved in the process as they were only trying to keep a broken system from going away. Sadly, that same system is moving civilization toward what we are now calling climate change. The New Jersey Supreme Court came to rule in favor of a judge ruling that a xerox copy of a paper had been "manufactured for trial purposes due to him not seeing any changes or erasures on the paper's surface." He would not allow a faculty member who had used that paper many years before, for its stated purpose, to testify to its lawful existence. The judge said he was done with testimony. To make his final decision he had added a word to the applicable state law so as to find me guilty of disobeying the law. He felt that word should have been there all alone.

The local newspaper, the Star Ledger of Newark, NJ, reported on the case where almost everything reported was inaccurate. The chief reporter promised me that she would let me review her reporting prior to publishing if I would remain calm and let her do her work. She never let me review any of her reports. When I later asked why she commented that she had been too busy. Thus, she kept a bad system alive.

> Clearly, the judge was acting as the agent of the university. From a NYC NPR report on the trial the CEO of foreign firm on the Fortune 500 list, that was on my management school's board, stated: "You American's are very skilled. You can pay judges on top of the table. Back home we must still do so under the table." (From a Luncheon with Businessmen in NYC)

The above experiences were essential to clarify the not so understandable processes involved in the US approach to environmental deterioration and attempted protection. Via what I had experienced on my farm and in Vietnam I had a special interpretation of the human role in climate change as I saw its early beginning in the nineteen seventies. This is the impending force that will define whether or not humans are fucked during the rest of this century. Much of the following book attempts to explain how this makes no sense (cents?) for life but made many dollars for a few humans.

Being a shit-fighter is not a particularly poetic nor attractive mission to carry out in life, but it does seem essential to manage many experiences of life. Many may find such as rude speak. Perhaps it is. My problem has been with the smell from many interaction rituals I was bought into, or trapped in, by society; that collection of social beings that seemed to have participated in the Faustian Dilemma, then negotiation, then sale of their soul for the cheap. If you find such concern a waste of your short life then please do not attempt to go into this book. You obviously have better things to do. I don't know what they are but let's hope you do, or your leadership will expose you to them.

Thirty episodes of Faustian negotiations in my life are outlined in the following where I failed to sell my long-term soul for short-term gain. Perhaps I was simply short-sighted, misinformed about the meaning of life, or not so intelligent. My soul meant much to me. Yes, at times it was a very heavy weight.

If your parents, or your grandchildren advise you to avoid this book please listen to them. They have good arguments against its content and for not looking it up in life. Being woke, or awake, can be an expensive posture in contemporary life. Pretending to be asleep prior to pretending to go to your private heaven is a more popular posture. As such your need to be popular and be valued as such is crucial to any who open this book. Any fight against shit can become very unpleasant in that you walk away with traces of the experience on you, if indeed you are able to walk away afterwards.

IV

METAPHORIC OR ACTUAL

"Humans are fucked," is an unsettling idea. It is especially irritating to those dedicated to climbing societal hierarchies via Maslow's "Hierarchy of Needs," as they think only the "low class" use such terms. It is not so far from plans to fuck others for self-esteem to becoming fucked by a looping behind. As will be explained herein, the long tradition of Faustian Bargaining as it was further developed via ideas of industrialization since 1850 now has much to unravel in its Faustian Tragedy. The process of which such is a part increasingly seems like a plan organized by what humans have long referenced as the devil.

In most schools, especially those motivating the individual to work, teaching of the hierarchy of leadership of work is central to the culture, its politics, its science, even its religion. The price is paid by the context, mostly the natural environment, that resources are taken from to fulfill the self. Meeting bio-needs more productively expands into defining and seeking psycho-wants about rooms and objects to place in them. Such explains an outline version of how a growing number of humans are feeling they are fucked. Perhaps we occupy the culture of the fucked.

1. Educated In The Metaphoric

Our education presumes a societal structure where meaning is supplied by a hierarchy of importance. Thus, we are encouraged to work ever harder to achieve access to ever more stuff. Piles of stuff thus become important, perhaps the focus of the culture is on piles of stuff. If you are not born at the top and see that you need to work ever-harder and ever-longer to do well, while avoiding the confusion of doing good, then you are easily angered upon hearing that humans, including you, are simply fucked by what you do and choose to not do.

To be fucked in a non-sexual sense is becoming interesting to examine. It is becoming an indicator of change in society, and possibly the world. As such it has many meanings that has evolved over the years. Its current means can help us understand much about humans and their changed context.

In the 16th century to be fucked was mostly to reference the complete negativity of the subject, not a reflective commentary about humans and their context. For 500 years the concept has broadened from sex linked to violence and/or pleasure then comment on being capable of such in Frisian, Dutch or German. The spelling of fuck began to be spread between languages yet used to insult people or represent sex, both as vulgar associations. During this entire course of history, until recently fuck was censored and controlled. The online *Etymology Dictionary* says it was seen as so insulting that it was seldom ever written down.

It was simply banned from the English dictionary from 1795 until 1965. Even as its banning would violate principles of free speech in places like America, they still attempted to ban swear words, even while such was becoming more common in many other places. In 1873 the US went so far as to make it illegal to print swear words in passing the Comstock Act. Printing fuck would put the writer in jail, even though the statute had no clear definition of obscenity. Before the end of the 19th century in America fuck was exclusively negative. By the end of the 20th century, it had come to mean much more. Just now psychological researchers encourage its widespread use as a stress reliever.

To better understand a context, one needs to reflect on the context of being human. If you believe you must climb ladders you will soon come to believe such must be done at any cost, even to the context. You soon believe you are important, even immortal. Thus, you learn to help yourself at any cost to the larger environment, i.e., the context of your life that includes others and nature.

Relative to how such humans shop, walk, drive, talk and listen, the more sexual sense of the concept is okay, but any attempt to see such more holistically brings irritation, even legal order consequences. Such humans were educated to believe effective leadership, by them or of them, comes from the shining lights of optimism.

2. Learning of the Actual

When teaching I made a distinction between education and learning, a difference that becomes very basic to life and your success in it. Most education is to encourage students to memorize answers to questions, where the questions are mostly unquestioned. Each lecture and most tests are set up to see how well the memorization went. My bias is quite different. I would encourage students to ask questions about most things, including me. Where the questions are good, the answers become more obvious and need not be memorized. Improved questions are seen to be the basis for improvement in education, society, and self. Questions relate to asking why we make such and such, not how to make it with more productivity as if it's obvious why such is necessary. Good CEOs learn this quickly in each company. Key to good questions is concern with what is then being done. Some call this questioning pessimism, but it's better than the later pessimism that will be deserved when you keep doing the wrong thing.

Ambrose Bierce, in his Devil's Dictionary of 1888, commented at length on the human condition and its contradictions with life. The one below is from his page 132 of an American Century

Addition of his book, as seen in a copy given to me by one of my great professors –

> Optimism. .*n.* The doctrine, or belief, that everything is beautiful, including what is ugly, everything good, especially the bad, and everything right that is wrong. It is held with greatest tenacity by those most accustomed to the mischance of falling into adversity and is most acceptably expounded with the grin that apes a smile. Being a blind faith, it is in accessible to the light of disproof – an intellectual disorder, yielding to no treatment but death. It is hereditary, but fortunately not contagious.

Perhaps it's not contagious yet we seem to look for leaders that represent our faults, and come to symbolize unsubstantiated optimism, especially when we are assured that we can later criticize them for being failures. Given the chance they hope to be that light. As such a social decorum must be maintained as defined by a particular culture that gives them shelter. They find "humans as fucked" to depressing for leadership and even too gross to think of, and especially wrong to state. None-the-less they were still born with a death certificate.

Those "up the hierarchy" of being human do exhibit a fear of change. They become leaders via a leadership agenda that attracts those with a similar phobia against the natural, against change as continuance. Noting that those with wealth tend to be protected from change, they "naturally" seek to accumulate wealth in a society via its cultural definition of the day. As they carry their certificate of death along each day of their life, they act to compose an empire of dirt. Even the dirt they are buried under is not long connected to them. Change rules, nature governs.

Herein life is defined as change, death as changelessness. If you are interested in this difference look into the human battlefield defined by Parmenides versus Heraclitus. They depend on a hierarchical separation to define their protection from the instability of change. They are protected from the cost of changelessness. I embrace ideas that can unsettle as they point to the price that must be paid by my environment and me to be sealed from change.

I see it as a bit tragic in that humans choose to be upset about losing what they didn't work for, don't have, and refuse to clarify relative to their moving into their future. The values initiate dangerous debates where the best results will be what eliminates the hierarchies they now depend upon. They fear they may fall lower in society ranking. They will regardless.

The stance taken herein is different. The hierarchy of you being above me, or humans being above other forms of life in our world is a problem for all of life. Thought to be a basis for arrogance of humans, such hierarchies become a cause of many problems in and of life. As we are now seeing the hierarchy of humans above all other forms of life is leading to climate change that destroys the context of life. As an Iowa farmer with cows roaming "freely" in my pastures, I fail to think well of my culture, what it locks up and consumes.

"Humans are fucked" is an invitation to a shockingly serious discussion about the conditions of life on our planet and to where life is heading based on human norms that denigration then deteriorate context. Life is clearly under threat. It faces non-existence from human behavior, especially that of the wealthiest in the richest societies. Those taking the most out from nature seem to be those who argue most strongly for decorum via traditional cultural norms. Those norms were mostly derived to maintain and protect a hierarchy of wealth. Its exhibition and the hierarchy required as a difference that fails to make a difference in support of life. It's the basis for mental slavery.

My concern for the above and its probable consequences is great. I sense it's already too late for innovative, even viable, responses to these threats. I researched this in the nineteen-seventies then wrote a book on it in 1979. That book was reprinted forty years later as: "Too Early, Too Late, Now what?"

The above is growing into the most important topic in nations, organizations, families, and the human mind. Even those wars that the masculine aspect of being human, to compensate for penis size (i.e., Putin, et.al.), seems trivial in comparison to human destruction of life's context. At the dinner table, youth are told they don't seem to want to work, they use regrettable language and appear to respond to a life not worth living via threats of suicide. In fact, they are very concerned about the conditions of their future life if they work as their parents did to maintain business as usual. The elderly that are most concerned with their legacy in death become very threatened with youthful discussions of graveyard urination ceremonies upon those that created the conditions making life uninhabitable. These are rather ugly dinners if they are even to be held anymore. Surely we can do better. Perhaps we begin by accepting we might well be fucked as an accurate state for the future.

In the first argument it is made clear, by the older, that rational discourse and thinking are essential values. To forego such will destroy the culture. Parents and teachers point out that certain expressions are helpful while others should not be allowed. The argument of the second is that a culture that has so destroyed the conditions of a context required by life needs to be destroyed. What is needed is access to a deeper level of questioning about what humans do. The path we are on as driven by the culture we have is taking us to conditions were life, via all species of it, is fucked. Surely humans can learn to do better, if better can be found.

Herein the culture that brings serious damage to the conditions of context that define and maintain life on our planet is deeply questioned. I attempt to define a present state of danger as well as outline a warning of even greater danger awaiting many forms of life, including human life. Perhaps I'm trying to bringing attention to myself, or to a simple-minded concern that has always been part of the backdrop of the human condition. Or perhaps I'm talking of a new and very dangerous to life context of life. Perhaps we are living in an early warning that something is wrong in human behavior organized around the ever more productive meeting of bio-needs and wider access to what might best be seen as psycho-wants. Perhaps the changes to context we are creating are beyond human capabilities in managing what it initiates. If so then we can ask are humans actually fucked?

Under debate for thousands of years such clearly ambiguous statements signify occasional concern for the status of some aspect of business as usual. Sometimes, as during a world war between humanly generated ideologies, it signifies an impending end state, as when two nuclear bombs were released upon Japan for failing to respect their unrespectful behavior towards non-Japanese. Can it be an alert to more widespread troubles as in a world war against mother nature via expanding the downside of father time?

The expanded use of we humans fucked has taken it as common knowledge into much of the experiencing of life. Even the context of life seems troubled. Humans are more urgently challenged by rapidly growing irregularities and threats to continuance. The idea of hurt is thus being expanded, perhaps beyond managerial capabilities throughout social situations against natural backdrops.

At an atmospheric level the comment suggests ambiguous clarity about a low point in the situation of being human. As one is drawn closer to the ground, as we now are despite our dreams of avoiding such, we encounter experiences that provide unavoidable information. Something is changing. "I love you very much but can't be near you anymore." Such provides entry into a context for our hearts where we clearly ask any who still listen: "What the fuck is going on here?" This is intended to include what we do, why we do it, and what seem to be the consequences of such?

With time humans learn to hurt then respond to hurt by spreading the it, or seeking to move up the hierarchy from sensing there is less hurt further up. Thus, we use hurts as an organizing force as well as our entry point into understanding why and from whom we are "being fucked." The two are related in that when we sense we are to be hurt, and its too late to avoid such, we soon realize we had been fucked. Via the consequences of climate change all humans will come to understand that it means to become fucked, and fucked due to our prior activities and values. Both concepts seem to thus be expanding at a personal and interpersonal level these days. If in doubt about this growth look at all forms of widely disseminated communication, e.g., in person, computerized, and phone use. We were not warned of this in those 1940's handbooks on the cybernetic-self and its potential to finally access negative entropy. Since then, entropy has only increased, and more are hurt more often. Our setting and its occupants seem to be fucked.

What should humans do? What are humans capable of doing related to the emerging hurt? We watch the older population seek increased stability and changelessness from the instability their prior actions initiated. We see how youth become increasingly upset with the stage having been set by those actions of their elders. Youth desperately seek change, at least in those what are older. Hurt within and between those groups grows. One group seems passionate to support the sayings of Parmenides in 4th Century BC Greece while the other stands on the ideas of 3rd Century BC Heraclitus. One wears the clothes of "changelessness," the other becomes more naked about the potentials in "change." Some adamantly argue that life shows how things only become worse via change. Others point out how change is essential to life, and any sort of future in its occupation. Both are limited but clearly speak from self-interest. Things are no longer what our leaders tell us, yet we are not yet willing to attempt self-leadership. Clues of the seriousness of this are seen in sharply increased suicide rates and seeing college attendance as not a dream.

Perhaps it is helpful to return to 1992 when REM composed and sang the song: "Everybody Hurts." It was organized as a very clear statement to teenagers who were contemplating suicide based on their view of their context and to where it seemed to be headed. It inspired me to work with a group of Lakota Indian youth that were very discouraged about their placement in mythology and land mass in the USA. They didn't see hope in elders being able to make it all better, or even fix parts of it. Thus, exit seemed like the best option.

In 2014, after being fired from a dean and then professor's job at New Jersey Institute of Technology I became overtly excited about the hope found whenever management says it's too late. That is when leadership that makes things seem bad becomes afraid of their responsibility and goes underground into hiding. According to a judge of part of the firing process NJIT should punish me for lack of respect for leadership but keep me as I would best help them survive their probable future. New Jersey's Governor of the day, Chris

Christie, was on the firing committee and lead them in the rule of leaderships with nowhere to go, thus proudly ignoring the judge's advice via much anger. The NJIT president that led the firing was encouraged to return to a job in Alabama where his arguments with David Hawk about being a racist was okay were easier acceptable. Then, three years later Christie captured an approval rating of 15%, the low for all NJ state governors.

During times of turbulence social interaction becomes unstable. Some argue this arises due to increased clarity, but I will instead argue that the societal stress comes from threats to the context of society and suggests major disruptions to human interaction and exchange with other humans and their context. Some might rise to claim this is caused by increasing evidence of climate change. I will instead argue that the situation is no longer one of cause-effect relations. In fact, such logic may well have provided the largely ignored threat to surface, expand and become dangerous. I will go on to argue that we are entering an age of "effects of effects" and not continuation of "cause-effect" management.

Humans frequently encounter, deal with, or use ideas related to expressions such as "fuck you," "fuck me," or as in this publication on threats to our world – "we are fucked." Such are encountered during our days in listening to others, or reflecting on ourselves, while life unfolds around us. "We Are Fucked" is somewhat special. It implies reflection on our status in this world and perhaps the next. Stated in small cases or emphasized in capitals, the expression and its punctuation vary via the hierarchy of human feelings. It can be followed by a coma, period, series of dots, question marks or even emphasized via an exclamation mark.

What follows is not to ignore those with closely held religious principles requiring public avoidance of sexual inuendoes that must be kept voiceless, such as religious fathers keeping pregnant daughters from abortions, or those finding silent no no's more exciting than open discourse on their meaning. This is intended to enhance open discussion of human predicaments and the role of humans in managing those they have created via their own efforts and the value systems that drive those efforts. Simply put, in the words of the terribly thoughtful song by REM – Everybody Hurts.

3. To Improve Business as Usual, Stop It

Humans invest much of life's effort to improve something, someone, or self. Via limited definitions of improvement much of what they invest can in fact make things worse, even threaten what they love and need. Herein I hope to address ideas for improvement in a different way, one that can accommodate a changing context. I will illustrate how many prior efforts to improve became major threats.

With much pride, limited knowledge, and little to no ethical clarification they seek improvement. Initiating the process, or emerging via it, these humans seek control or seem to desire to be closely aligned with it. With limited intelligence, no ethical certainty, and limited care for context they continue. There is little to no reflection on the environment, or of anything beyond a tight focus on individualized missions.

Expenses from self-centered activities are given little thought. Costs to context and bystanders are mostly ignored. Such seems to be the current definition of human beings being human. Not only do leaders act this way but followers tend to be attracted to leadership with such characteristics, e.g., leaders going nowhere. If we have no appreciation of our context then why not accept offers of leadership from a similar absence of knowledge and caring for the good. If you are dumb and/or bad why not go for similar qualities in leadership illustrating the importance of leadership with nowhere to go.

Many respond with so what, why not or go away. Some say humans are a transient species with more potential than intelligence so hang on for better, or absence of anything.

Sometimes there is no improvement, even where the need is very great. The future cost of such can be catastrophic just as it is seen to be too late to change for the necessary improvement. At the present time this is coming to appear as consequences fateful to those initiating them and not results from results as noted and filed away.

We even see greater evidence of efforts to improve as becoming counterproductive. As such, conditions worsen.

Human efforts begin in thoughts about the meeting of bioneeds and psych-wants. With time the action from such thinking often loses its way. As such humans have learned to distance themselves from any causal role in a downward headed process, but in so doing humans ignore the chance to manage such activities better. Egotism seems to be a central attribute to understanding human conduct. As noted in the 1911 Devil's Dictionary:

> "Egotist – A noun, as a person of low taste, more interested in himself than in me."

In essence the causes and effects become difficult to connect and impossible to understand context from. A clue to this being part of a threatening situation is where the results of prior mistakes are described as consequences, not bad results from bad actions. We therein see a connection purposefully broken between the initiator and thus responsibility is avoided. An indication that this is occurring in a family, organization or nation is seen in the history of a group of followers reverently praising the amazing skills of a dysfunctional leader. In such instances who is being blamed for the wrongdoing? Many books on the decline of social organizations, especially companies and nation states, provide insights into this question. This is clearly seen in the history of leadership by such personalities as Catherine the Great, Joseph Stalin, Adolf Hitler, Mussolini, Mao Zedong, King Leopold II, Pol Pot, Vladimir Putin, and Donald Trump.

Once disconnected from the initiator of a problem we then must find the proverbial cause. We humans often begin with the concept of nature. We point out how she, once again, stood in the way of or simply failed to cooperate with her highest achievement – men. She comes to be seen as the enemy of manly progress. As the plot of a tragedy unfolds we have trouble not seeing that somehow men were involved in creating the mess, or at least took a role in worsening it. We then look around us to find who could have done such. This is where the major conflict with others and nature begins. We see where other men something did to displease us before and thus when it reappears, we exaggerate it. Lacking such we point to a natural phenomenon that disturbed or even destroyed out context. If we remain conscious we might eventually see how some of this bad was a result of our own prior acts. That is to be avoided at all costs, if we are on a happiness trek, but sometimes the mirror is too clear to ignore. The focus herein is making better use of the mirror and the information available in it.

We undertake efforts to improve the conditions for humans yet many prove to be counterproductive to the concern for life on earth. The initial concern and their responses now form a composite seeming to collectively endanger life more deeply. Is there a way for humans to change this negative process? Such can bring the power of hope to provide a meaningful basis for life, and definition to its meaning. The alternative is not very inviting, as the book's title should imply.

Under industrial conditions humans came to act in ways that eroded life's essential conditions. Some conditions are on an eradication timetable. Discussion of the why and how such could happen requires more room than allowed herein, but at least we can seek a better foundation for the human project on this planet. Key is coming to appreciate the basis of life, herein defined as its context. Environment includes all that appears to surround the object in question.

Context is more specific than environment thus encourages more beneficial action. Both envelop a subject, but context allows focus on characteristics of a subject and how best to manage or improve those characteristics and not say "its complex, complicated and out there beyond me." Many use the two interchangeably and thus end with muddled ambiguity. When confronting issues of life, including its continuance, it is helpful to focus on that which we interact with. This can even include those interaction rituals, called culture, which we rely on to give definition to who and what we are.

Context includes the stores we stop in on the way home in our car to buy presents that no one needs, nor likes, to reassure others and our self that we matter became they do. Driving to, picking up, and buying a card, a bottle of wine, and then presenting it works to keep a situation, a relationship, as it has been, i.e., changeless, even if it must change. Walking home, kissing, and hugging your best friend, saying you feel a need to change then ask: "Please, can you help me?" is more natural, graciously meaningful, and hopeful.

My objective herein is to study the interaction rituals, even fights, with ourselves thus avoid the expensive interactions with others, and/or nature. As will be noted later, farmers alone on their tractors often discover the first while thinking of the second and third. Erwin Goffman was very helpful in describing the process for discovering ourselves in *The Presentation of Self in Everyday Life* in 1959. Many problems we face in our context, and our environments, are derived from the difficulties outlined in Goffman's work.

Just now the conditions underlying context are unstable and begin to defy life. Questions grow relative to available energy sources, minerals key to essential making of products, and plants to support life and/or nourish it. Just now air and water qualities and weather conditions required of life are moving outside essential limits. The traditional stability required for life's continuance is moving. Planetary life seems endangered by the context that it once found security from and nourishment in. Dangers to systems of life expand consistent with changing updates from science. Most humans seem to not care, even the few that understand. Is it harsh to say, "humans are fucked."

Contextual dangers are growing in severity, more than ever experienced in human history on Earth. The future threats range from indirectly created devastating storms to directly caused nuclear warfare. There is irony in both types of danger to life. The conclusion is clear that human activities are a major threat to life, including that of humans. The clearest conclusion seems to be that humans are totally fucked. This may seem as totally beyond rude inside the need for clarity.

My advice is to move deeper and wider into the shit in how humans have become responsible for all of the above. While reflecting you may begin to see that your fear of rudeness is a trivial concern. Yes, there is now a growth in societal rudeness and an expansion of the traditional disharmony in and between humans.

Instead of going deeper into the value systems that define and manage what humans do and how they do it we often stay in the superficial. Instead of seeing from where the hate and fear comes we comment that "The times are difficult." From this opening we describe how climate has always been defined by change and we should trust it will change for the better. We advise each other that we need to avoid thinking so pessimistically about the potential that humans are fucked. Instead we need to calm down and trust that it will be okay in the future. If it's too late then why should we worry about it. As with the closing scene of "Don't Look Up, we should throw a nice dinner party for those we like being around. Things, including humans, come and go thus what's the big deal? Humans take great pride in not being very smart. Perhaps ignorance is a strong base for pride?

The conception of fucked as used here avoids the pleasant pathways open to foreplay within a dinner fest just prior to sexual intercourse, or as an entrée to a more interesting web conversation that was dying out. Herein it reflects on the downside of a species, not two individuals in search of deeper meaning, as the species heads into a bad ending. Many of you may find the image of our species heading into an end-state upsetting, but you will probably find life fading even more upsetting.

Improvement in the human pathway towards meaning that borders on relevance will seem to require change in how humans do what they do, and change in how they arrive at the values sponsoring it. We might look at fuck in a euphemistic[25] manner, and not as literal as marketed in porno movies. This will take us deeper in seeking and finding suitable business as unusual, and ways to bypass the limitations now seen in business as usual. At first look this would seem to call for inclusion of the more systemic processes of seeing

---

[25] One of my favorite professors at the University of Pennsylvania, and good friend, Russell Ackoff dedicated one of his many business management books to me with a note I will never understand: "To David Hawk, who was euphemistically called a 'student'."

and thinking, as used by those studying the cosmos, and thinking of the science of physics at the edge. This is very different from the Greek tradition of being educated to become fixated on the analytic gained from reductionism, and the limitations associated with such. The Greek tradition was clearly grounded in the homocentric, with a few exceptions who found no meaning in no context. For them, context required appreciation of life as dynamically linked to conditions essential to its continuance. Now in the 21st Century we begin to see what bothered them about the rationality of the analytic.

To see the difference more clearly we need rise above those strange hierarchies of subjects that allowed for self-importance. Such led to belief in being able to discover immortality trips via funded research based on directed optimism. To get funding they must in some way avoid or discount ideas of universally imposed mortality on the researchers and their supervisors. Later in this book we will go into the human bias towards discovery and selling of "negative entropy" as to be found in science and technology and thus advertised on all TVs and cameras even when not found.

V

LEARNING FROM THOSE WHO
NEED TO FUCK ME UP, OR OVER

- One reviewer asked how can a former professor, dean, university scholar with four degrees, with three Ivy league, find fuck to be acceptable distinction to make use of?
- Another wanted to know if CEOs I advise find my behavior acceptable.
- A third accused me of talking like a farmer. I thanked him. He responded - "Hmmm."

At a higher level of discourse the question could be: "How wrong must things be to justify use of such a term?" Maybe I have an egocentric need to transcend societal values and discourse? Perhaps I was demonstrating the downside of one of the many insights offered by Ambrose Bierce back in 1881 is his attempt at defining human limitations from thinking they are great. His definition of Egotist is informative to our age, as seen in his Devils Dictionary. It implies something of the content of the book and author intended in some humor, but perhaps seeming to focused on the author?

The metaphor for my life beginning at an early age was: "It's the fight against shit. That's what it's all about." Your response should be how can Hawk be so rude and vulgar? Settle down, it will get worse.

Was that funny? The following notes provide a brief outline of how being a shit fighter comes to be a creed for surviving life in a series of difficult environments. Many of my close friends experienced worse environments than those I will depict, but many of them had learned to accept the unacceptable. These included many close friends such as David Williams, a close friend student at Iowa State University. in which I lived. Others have had a much more difficult pathway, but I would not recommend mine or theirs as a desirable pathway to death. On the following pages the low/high points of life are presented as sketches. Others, that were present at each of these situations might have different recall but that is for them to struggle with.

1. In The Beginning: There Was Nothing

1944 – Born at home. Our farm was ten miles away from the hospital with a gravel road that was often in bad shape connecting the two. Mother said my arrival was easier than that of my older brother two years prior. She went to the hospital afterwards just in case.

1948 – While helping plant the family garden at age four I commented that it was strange to plant in such non-natural ways, with single varieties placed in long straight rows. Nature seemed to do better with arrays of species, diversity, in more natural arrangements. My dad sent me to the farmhouse. He said something was fucked about my attitude; thus I was a nuisance to necessary work. (A gifted scientist Stuart Kauffman, and I hope friend, would come to explain the crucial importance of variety in keeping nature alive.)

1950 – I was sexually molested at age five. It was by a very conservative and religious uncle. This happened while I was living with my grandmother, so I told her about her son's need to hurt. She asked me to not worry about such and move on with my life. To elaborate she said her son was troubled and involved in difficult discussions with God. She said once those were done God would make it all better. As such I learned to avoid grandmother and her son as much as possible.

I came to presume he was simply a selfish idiot, like many religious conservatives I came to know in Iowa. I thus recommended he stay with cows for his earthly delights as they didn't seem to notice what he was up to. Yes, I had been fucked.

1951-1955 – Each Sunday, from age six my brother and I were driven to Sunday School then Church by a great uncle, no, not the one with the sex problem with his God. This was a much older uncle that picked us up at home and then drove us to church. He was a sheep farmer but not so good. He would often have a dead sheep on the floor of the back seat or in his trunk. I mention this because he seldom disposed of them in a timely manner and after a few days the smell would test anyone's tolerance for what shouldn't be. He lives with his sister. I was told that on occasions she would use them in cooking, which was probably why it was said that no one, absolutely no one, would eat at their home. If my brother would comment on the smells and insects running around on the carcass the uncle would respond: "Just be quiet. It's part of life." Thinking we were experiencing the aftereffects of death, not life, we thus avoided talking to him. Family?

1956 – Our house had no indoor plumbing thus we had an outhouse for toilet needs just behind the house. When I was twelve I was using what was affectionately called the shithouse when my brother leaned a wooden beam with a spike in it against the door. The spike hit my head when I opened the door. About 4-inches of it went through my cheek into my jaw. We could not seem to get it out thus we walked to an uncles' house; yes, another uncle. My brother carried the beam and I walked beside him. Seeing the uncle we asked him to please drive us to a doctor to stop the pain. Upon seeing us, the uncle simply ignored me and the spike in my head and ran after my brother. When he caught him he beat him. When done he explained that there are priorities in life, and I should take note of "first things first." I did not understand why humans need to fix a cause before an effect. The uncle drove me to town to a doctor, who removed the "effect." I felt fucked.

1957 – When I was thirteen my brother and I were ordered to sit in front of the church congregation in a formal ceremony just for us. We had been charged with blasphemy and abusing Sunday School teachers with our not very funny questions. Some examples were: "Is God a woman?"/ "Was Jesus, with 12 boyfriends, Gay?"/ "Is it okay to be mean as hell if you are a Christian, then ask forgiveness at heaven's gate?" We were found guilty and never allowed in that church again. Actually, that was nice for our futures.

2. Continuation: Signs of Something

1961 – Elected President of my local high school Future Farmers of America Chapter. My first act was to criticize the school management. Farm students were to help the community by killing pests, varmints, and rodents then bring evidence of the killing via heads, tails, or legs to the front desk of school. This was proof of our work success. Some appeared similar to house pets, but I was told that they too can be pests. I got students to protest the endeavor and thus suspend it while I was president. School management was upset with me. I was thus punished and banned from taking college preparatory math or English courses until graduation. I instead read books on the subject. They thought they were fucking me over.

1962 – As FFA President I protested the county watershed commission planning to cut down an old tree that was often filled with birds. The tree was thought to interrupt the flow of the adjacent stream taking water to a river. The country authorities wanted water to run away more rapidly. I thus embarrassed the country commission by showing the science of their being mistaken. The Izsak Walton League of America helped me then gave me the award for the year in keeping the tree alive for birds and allowing the stream to behave naturally. I was regularly beat up at school by boys that were sons of the commission members. They informed me that what needed to move, the stream, needed to move faster. Trees must go away, and the job of birds was to fly, not hang out in trees. I learned much from them while being beaten.

1963 – I decided to go to college to see if life could be different. My uncle, the one who enjoyed beating my brother, advised me to not go to Iowa State University and if there never to study electrical engineering. He said ISU was the best university in the nation and EE was the hardest subject to study at ISU. Since he was wrong about most things in life, I had no choice thus I went to ISU and studied electrical engineering.

I had been responsible for milking 20 to 30 Jersey cows' morning and night for more than a decade. Then, during each day, I was to help with farming. My father was very angry about me leaving for college and thus no longer milking his 26 cows each morning and night. My family was quite poor thus I worked nights to pay for food, rent and tuition. My best job was for UPS in Des Moines loading and unloading trucks from 8 PM until 4 AM each night.

My course work suffered a bit from all this, but I had no choice relative to funding my schooling. I was seen as troublesome in my classes as I had read extensively on the subjects before university. In my first physics class I interrupted the lecturer and asked if we could also discuss entropy and its relation to negative entropy. He threatened to ban me from the class if I mentioned such again. I thus assumed I was on to something important. Regardless of exam grades he gave me a D.

3. Continuing: Seeing More of Something

1966 – I had been drafted by a local draft board due to my changing my degree program from a four to a five-year degree, as well as demonstrating against national ethics of invading Vietnam. I did say fuck you to the draft board in response to their threat to punish me for changing my degree program. They immediately drafted me to report in two weeks to Ft. Leonard Wood, Missouri to learn the basics of efficiently killing others then onto Ft. Eustis, Va. to use helicopters to aid such killing.

1968 – As I was loading dead and wounded into my helicopter, I was ordered by a Captain to stop such and instead shoot at fleeing women and children. I suggested that I should instead shoot him. A hearing was then held under battle-field conditions to set an example for others as to the price of disobedience to an officer during battle. I restricted my defense to:

> "We the unwilling, led by the unqualified, to kill the unfortunate, die for the ungrateful."

After two hours it was recommended that I be promoted for my attitude while the Captain would be demoted for his. Two weeks later the Captain died via a bullet wound to the back of his head. My above statement came to be used by many in the seventies to them protest against our government being unwelcome to save Vietnam from itself while helping it be as bad as the US was.

I liked Vietnam very much and wanted to stay thus had signed up for extension of my stay until discharge. After 17 months I was discharged and sent home regardless of my wishes.

1969 – Returned to Iowa State University to complete my Architectural Engineering degree. Didn't like the stories from the professors so I arranged for a student group to go study in Merida, Yucatán to study Mayan archeology and architecture for the semester. The next year I arranged for a similar group of fellow students to study in Europe by hiring faculty there and arranging for students to live in homes for free. We were poor. Both study groups did very well.

1971 – The ISU faculty were less than happy with me and what I had done as a student. At graduation they awarded me: "The Scariest

Student in Engineering." I then returned to Germany to work for the architect I had hired to teach the students that was in the competition for designing the Olympic Games Site. I work with him on the project. He won then recommended me for a job in London working for the government body – Westminster City Council.

4. Culture: Reality as Continuation of The Usual

1972 – Managed several city design and building construction projects in central London. Once worked with a Margaret Thatcher, then Minister of Education, on a school design project in a housing community. I wanted it nice, she wanted it to look like a poor school, to motivate them to work harder. She ended up firing me from the project. I then took over a project to redesign and rebuild Piccadilly Circus, so cars could travel faster through it. I genuinely disliked it but was ordered to support it as a government employee. I then hired Edmund Bacon, from the University of Pennsylvania, to be an advisor on the project. He was great. I arranged to have the project halted via Bacon's advice. I was fired. Professor Bacon then invited me to be his teaching assistant at Penn. In much respect for him I thus moved to Philadelphia.

1973 – After one semester of architecture courses at Penn I was asked by the Chair to please avoid courses in architecture. I was told I could look elsewhere and find credits to use for an architecture degree that I would be given. I did so. I met many remarkable teachers in many schools at the university including Engineering, the Annenberg School, and the Wharton School. They each taught me so very much about unforgettable subjects. Simultaneously I worked on a joint degree in City Planning with my 1974 thesis as – "The Communication Alternative: From moving concrete to moving ideas." It was to rethink cities, to get humans out of cars to walk around a city built around ideas travelling on electronic communications as society. I had a chapter on how if couples would date on machines, but never meet, there would be fewer divorces. The

Planning faculty flunked me in anger. Two of the leading faculty else-where in the university came to meet with the City Planning faculty to argue for study of my seemingly wild ideas. Those faculty thus changed the thesis grade to an A. Later in life I regretted the thesis on info tech. It was overtly optimistic about humans and the machines they create. Info-tech can to be seen as an unsuccessful replacement to automobiles.

1974 – Once those two professors got me a passing grade, they invited me to be their first student in a new PhD Program at Penn, to be called Systems Sciences and to be in the Wharton School. I was very happy to work with them and have their support. I was given a research and teaching assistantship to pay my costs in the school and not need to continue to work outside the university.

5. Challenging the Usual

1975 – I left Philadelphia to move to Stockholm to work at the School of Economics as a teacher and to establish a new research center, the Institute of International Business at the Stockholm School. Two friends, Lars Otterbeck and Gunnar Hedlund, allowed me to help set up the Institute, called IIB. We attracted many students and millions of dollars to a research center that could reflect on many dimensions of future business. I was allowed to articulate and propose Its first research venture: "Environmental Deterioration: Analytic Solutions in Search of Synthetic Problems." It was to study the international deterioration of nature by business activities. It involved 20 major firms and 6 governments in the world. In the end it concentrated on 10 companies having production in two countries. One conclusion was that regulation would not control human pollution but failure to do so would end in conditions of climate change that would ter-minate most species.

A major scientist at Exxon, Dr. Black, taught me about the science of climate change. He also taught me about the first human to discover in 1856 how human-centered industrialization would create climate change. She had been a farm girl descendant from the Isaac Newton family. Her name was Eunice Newton Foote. The CEOs of Exxon and Texaco became heavily involved in the research and both later began to lecture on its results, before being replaced by their Boards with men that would support the dark side of energy accessibility.

1977 – Sweden's Prime Minister presented the results of the IIB Project to OECD where the Chair of my Systems Sciences Program at Penn read of it. He called me and told me I had completed my PhD with that work. Another professor said climate change research was my conclusion, but he wanted to know more in a dissertation of how humans should manage the consequences. I trusted him and wrote 256 pages on what humans should do to manage climate change.

6. One More Time: Business-as-Usual Management

1978 – The dissertation, including the three volumes of the research conclusions and the one additional volume of what humans needed to do passed after two years of difficult review. The Dean of Wharton was upset with the project, its conclusions and theory for how business as usual needed to be changed. His note to me argued that climate change was a hoax. He never talked to me again. The Director of the US EPA collected all copies of my reports that could be found in EPA offices and sent them to my Iowa farm with a quite angry cover letter about climate change as "junk science." My fellow students were so impressed by such leadership that they had my dissertation published by the University in 1979 titled: *Regulation of Environmental Deterioration.* #79-12. Key to it was the following thesis:

Much of mankind's history is written with regard to the successes of respective modes of social regulation. Although considerable individual achievement can take place during 'turbulent' times, when social regulation has failed, it is here assumed that greater achievements are possible when social regulation provides for a minimum stability so that interactions might have continuity and longer-term meaning. This assumption is in line with the central thought behind a Chinese curse: 'May you live in interesting times.' Stabilized human interaction allows potential for enough uncertainty, without that induced by the movement of the ground beneath the situation as well.

There are many modes available for man to regulate a situation's ambiguity, but each tends to contain its own destabilizing forces. This is in part due to how the regulation mode accommodates natural change which occurs in all situations, and in part due to the inherent potential for changing a situation as contained by each human actor. Continuation of our present model of regulation will create extremely destabilizing conditions that may come to be called climate change consequences by 2030.[26]

1979 – While back on my Iowa farm I was contacted by the Dean, School of Design at Iowa State University. He had read about my humorous history as a student at ISU and thus asked the faculty about me returning as a member of the faculty. Four leading professors threatened to resign if I was allowed to teach in "their" school. The Dean told me about this and said it is thus crucial to the student's future that I return to ISU. I should briefly teach while encouraging those who threaten to leave to do so. I took his offer for $17,500/year, while continuing to manage and work on the farm. Those professors were involved in my being given the "Scariest Student Award" at my graduation in 1971, a ceremony I had skipped.

1980 – I began an international program for students to travel abroad and bring faculty from other counties to lecture at Iowa State. Students took over its management. I then taught an architecture design studio. The course focused on building design for conditions

[26] David L Hawk, "S³ Papers: Regulation of Environmental Deterioration," Philadelphia, Pa: Social Systems Sciences, The Wharton School, University of Pennsylvania. 1979, pp. 1-2.

of climate change. We were in a newly built design center at ISU. It was a stretched skin glass building with no operable windows. Leadership thought an environment sealed from nature would give a technically sophisticated image. One night three of my students removed one of the large sheets of glass and filled the opening with Pella Double Hung windows. They argued cross ventilation was better for life and consumed less energy and avoided climate change. The fury in leadership and maintenance was great. The three students were removed from the university, but then awarded scholarships to the University of Pennsylvania. The remaining students in the class built a house of the future, as protest, behind the Design Center. It ended up as a three-story structure of soybean straw bales with a wooden structure. I was fired. The building basis for climate change conditions thus was continued.

7. Teaching As a Way To Learn About Change

1981 – I was offered a job in Boston at the Boston Consulting Group and teaching one class each year with a colleague at Harvard. He was from the Wharton School. The pay was to be $81,000/year plus Harvard pay. Upon hearing this the former Dean of the ISU school invited me down to visit a school in Newark where he had become Dean. I respected him and thus agreed to visit. Knowing me he had me meet with students, not faculty nor university's leadership. I loved the students and was willing to be there without a wage. He arranged for me to get $30,000/year. My response was a happy yes. (Later it turned out to be $27,500, but who keeps track of such.)

1982 – Became Associate Dean of Architecture. Designed two new degree programs, to link science to aesthetics, as well as got 247 new courses approved for the school to enhance the school's status for accreditation.

1983 – Worked with New Jersey's Governor via a research project into the limits from attempted regulation of the built environment.

I identified an uninhabited section of Newark NJ and proposed to turn it into a regulation-free zone, to see what business would do. This was to show human behavior if not regulated by politicians, lawyers, and angry officials paid to resolve conflicts by generating conflicts. 40 companies signed up to build projects in the zone, to show what they had long aspired to do. In 1986 it needed to be interrupted by my return to Sweden.

1987 – The project was interrupted by needing to return to my former work in Stockholm. A project I had once proposed needed to be initiated and then managed. It took two years followed by a seminar. At the seminar/conference the CEOs of 60 major international companies described their approach to managing in an unstable future. The subject was construction industry futures, with emphasis on design and building of infrastructures during destabilizing conditions such as climate change. It was titled "Conditions of Success" and cost $1 million.

1990 – I returned to the New Jersey school to teach and continue with my regulation free zone project. While gone another professor worked to use the project for other purposes by moving it to Atlantic City. An architect working for Donald Trump, as well as teacher, he wanted to shift the regulation free project to a site where Trump planned on building an Atlantic City Casino. They presumed being regulation-free would allow for cheaper construction. I thus arranged to meet with the architect then learned he had arranged for building maintenance to let him into my school office. He was searching for names of the 40 firms that were to have been involved. I had taken the list with me to Sweden and kept their interest alive while in Sweden. Somehow a client of his, a Donald Trump, had heard of my research on a regulation free zone and he wanted to have such for an Atlantic City Casino. I met the architect, then met with "The Donald" to discuss such. I found their attitude to be a problem. From those meetings Governor Kean and I stopped the project and returned the funding to state coffers.

1996 – My friend in life, Gunnar Hedlund, died. He had founded the Institute of International Business research center in Stockholm that I was a part of until his death. The replacement Institute Director then fired me at the funeral saying the Institute was not interested in issues related to environment, climate change, and all that "funny" stuff that Gunnar and I thought would reshape future business. Once Gunnar was gone the administration of the Stockholm School happily replaced Institute Board members and then assumed control of the considerable resources in the Institute's endowment. The new Director, who authored a textbook with the lead Professor of the Harvard B School then linked more of the Institute to Harvard. Gunnar and I had humorously rejected such for a long time. We felt Harvard was wedded to ideas in business as usual. Before long, interest in IIB went away and the Institute closed.

1998 –Began a project to build a different kind of research facility in a different way on my Iowa farm. It was to illustrate a new way, beginning with a 1918 Sears and Roebuck Craftsman House that was almost gone. Two neighbors as craftsmen helped me build the new place along with my fourth wife who was project manager. The project conditions were no timetable, no budget, no plans, no designation of space use prior to creating them, and using only 2 x 6 construction, triple pain windows, heavy insulation, geo-thermal heating and cooling, and natural materials. We ended with 8,000 square feet, four stories of spaces where we assigned uses after completion. It serves as the headquarters for many projects from many companies, requires almost no energy, is mostly composed of wood and tiles, and sees many visitors. Has six bedrooms, six bathrooms and six private studies. Nice place.

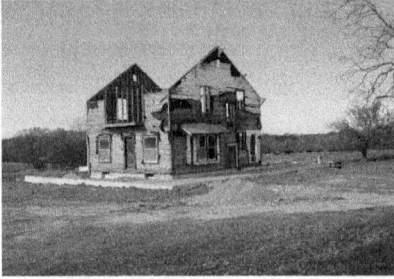

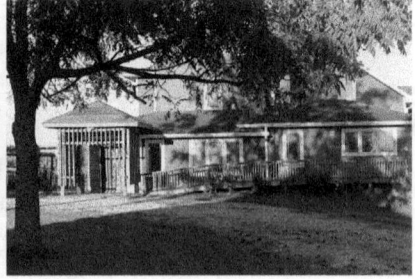

From the Dark   Inspired in the Light

1999 – Given the NJIT Alumni Association's Most Memorable Instructor Award. This came from a survey of students who graduated five or more years before from NJIT. A large reception was held in the university auditorium, but I was not listed as a speaker on the program, only the receiver of the main award. When handed the award the alumni yelled "speech." Thus, the university president asked me to say a few words, but without my normal FUs. From my respect for his leadership I only used FUs twice in my lecture.

Awarded the IBM International Professor of the Year Prize. Prior to this I had helped write a guidebook for the CEO of IBM on how this organization should best prepare for an unstable future. Open-Source approaches to computerization were key. IBM should let Google and Microsoft privatize their customers into anger, then government control, then let the Chinese pursue the open-source alternative to innovation after 2030. There was considerable money attached to the award, that I dedicated to student tuition payment. NJIT instead used the money for my salary, so my normal salary money could go to other uses. Secretaries secretly showed me how that happened where there was no light.

8. Test-Run As a Different Kind of "Leader"

2005 – Asked by a new NJIT Provost to serve as Acting Dean of the newly created business school at NJIT, one that was not doing well and in danger of the Trustees closing it. I gave up a job I had agreed to in Beijing as head of a Leadership Project at Tsinghua University but in respect to students of NJIT I agreed to the Dean's job for a year. Brought heads of several Fortune 500 firms, including the president of the number 12 firm and Chief of Staff of the number 6 firm, to be on the School's Advisory Board. I then made students responsible for designing new programs with the Advisory Board for their collective futures. I accepted the role of actual dean during a second year of service.

2005 – Faculty felt left out but based on their lack of attendance in School meetings and their bad treatment of students I began to feel they wanted to be left out. The School then became highly reaccredited and then awarded "The Most Improved Business School in North America." Four hours later NJIT's president fired me. He said I left him out of being credited with what I was doing. He was right.

2008 – In a Dean's meeting he became sufficiently angry with me to bring 8 charges against me as samples of illegal behavior. No guilt was found for any of the eight.

9. Learning: Why Leadership is of Changelessness

2009 – The president hired outside council and arranged to "pay a judge" to evaluation me for eighteen months of hearings. The judge, later called "NJIT's agent," found me to be guilty of one of the 25 charges. I then became distinguished in the regional press as the only tenured professor to be fired in the 136-year history of the university. A NYC newspaper had a headline: "NJIT strips tenure and fires professor for first time in school history." Oct 04, 2013. A Newark paper said:

> NJIT accused Hawk of abusing his power as dean, hiring a woman he lived with for a job and changing a business colleague's grade from an "F" to an "A," according to legal documents.

In fact Hawk's wife had invited the woman to stay at their house when she came for a job interview from Europe. Hawk's wife was originally from Europe. On the witness stand the judge asked Hawk's wife if she had permission from Hawk to invite the woman to stay with them? The wife's humble and noteworthy response was: "I wasn't aware I needed his permission." Later NJ judges turned that small weekend stay into "..she lived with Hawk…" Weak legal processes tend to capture the weaknesses that they attempt to obscure, consistently.

2011 – The process became a private research project into university crackage. Notes from the legal cases provide additional support to my seventies research that found legalisms and limitations of American trained lawyers advanced climate change while the lawyers sought more money. A group of companies I advised paid my legal cost for the five years spent in five courts, including New Jersey's Supreme Court. In the end, after the hearings were all concluded, the judge had to "modify" the relevant law on public servants. A friend of his on the Supreme Court later formally concurred that he carried such esteem that he could change a law in New Jersey. In response, the companies paying my legal costs stopped investing and expanding in New Jersey until there was new leadership in the state. Those "cracks" in the system.

Except for student tuition paying more than $5 million of the university legal costs to get even with Hawk the process was as humorous as it was informative One charge against Hawk was that his resume was dishonest as it left off some of the scholarly science papers he had published and some of the major research ventures he had created and attracted funding for. While they had never seen a professor do such, it truly was "dishonest" to whoever was seeking dishonesty in others. In addition, Hawk was charged with "stealing" state resources by submitting a bill for using the contents of his refreshment cabinet in his hotel room in Beijing. One night he had consumed $415 of alcohol, seemingly emptying the cabinet to become drunk.

The judge then asked to see the original receipts from NJIT since Hawk was not privy to them. When the judge saw them, he commented that it said 315, not 415, and was in Yuan, not dollars. This meant the reimbursement was a fraction of the amount in the charge. NJIT's legal counsel continued to argue that "The 415 was in dollars as the whole world uses dollars. Besides it was an American hotel thus if of course would use dollars. Besides, what are those Yuan's anyway?" The judge then said, "Now I understand, can we please move on from this?" This had been informative of NJ lawyers and law. Hawk seemed fucked.

> The collection of companies that were paying for Hawk's $1 million in legal costs felt they had learned much. They suspended their investment in New Jersey for a number of years. A later governor commented that I had fucked NJ.

2015 – Launched a new foundation in China as can still be seen on the EternalFeminine.org website. It was founded in 2015 to commemorate Donald Trump becoming leader of the US. It was to prepare the feminine to assume leadership in the near future, after humans could see how Donald would fail to reduce the suffering from climate change consequences as initiated by men via their managed industrial. The foundation theme was management was the major problem behind an approaching crisis for the planet, where the first three letters of management needed to be replaced. It was to train a new kind of leader in values of the feminine, to be known as "Femagement." The Foundation attracted $650 million in support in its first six months. The funding mostly came from leading Chinese businessmen who only had daughters, no sons. The Foundation was formally closed in 2021 by the government. China's leader felt China needed more masculinity to assume a stronger position in the world, not less power as implied by the feminine.

10. Helping Humans Learn Of Climate Change:

2018 – Began writing and publishing a series of books.

2020 – Began giving a series of Zoom and Skype lectures due to not being able to travel during Covid.

2023 – Continuing to write books while helping my sister Rachel with our Iowa farm. She and I are looking for better ways to produce food for the upcoming tragedies associated with temperature extremes, summer droughts, winter storms, and with too much industrialization in food production.

Absent landlords that don't know much about the land, nor care what it is, are also a problem. It is now a happy time on the farm. Last July it was plus 100 F, with no rain for 6 weeks. In January and February of this year it was minus 50 F with a wind chill factor. Next year the situation is to be even more unstable for life.

VI

ENTROPIC TRUTHS

Much of this book comes from the contents of *Sorry, Humans are Fucked*. Authored by "Hawkeye" it sold well but comments about it seem to focus on the title not content. Amazon banned it from their books but sold it as a "candle." I complemented them on their foresight in placement. "Next to candles your buyers can burn the book if they are frustrated with the contents." Management then sent it to T-shirts with dirty words on them. It sold well there also but reviewers suggested reprinting the book and dropping "that word," or at least a letter from it. They felt this would increase its appeal: "Sorry, Humans are Fucked." Oh well, that was the norm yesterday, not today.

1. Beyond Cause-Effect To Effects of Effects

The contents explain how ongoing human values and their associated actions guaranteed widespread hardship and increased mortality. Such reflections were avoided by most Americans. Americans were taught to await technological fixes to human problems and even dreams of discovery of negative entropy. This is seen in the work of Indrajit Samarajiva. He offered a recent review of "How, Precisely, We're Fucked: A Review of a seminal collapse textbook." He talked of a growing societal backlash against "Domers," perhaps even harsher than what was seen from those "workers" that republican "jokers" wage war against. Those seen as "woke" seemed more concerned about what humans were doing in becoming who they are than going shopping and enjoying life as long as it lasted. They criticized humans for accepting "gloom," not "bloom." My take on such distinctions will be what follows. Those arguing for "sleeping" as distinct from "waking" might only be joking?

From experience with humans at war with other humans and with nature my answer is simply – yes, humans are fucked. It was not reassuring to watch humans killing humans who failed to run away fast enough in Vietnam, all justified by shooters "protecting democracy" or "protecting their country." Women and children mostly thought of staying alive.[27] Later, in academic research I looked into the downside of production of products unworthy of use then dumped into the waste accepting natural lands. It was as disheartening as life in Vietnam. From watching such activities, it was hard to see hope in all those half-full glasses.

Humans killing each other, based on differences that weren't different, then carrying out a war of industrialization against nature, mostly to create what is ugly and in opposition to life, is hard to tolerate. The war against other is mostly left undiscussed herein although our war with ourselves is mentioned relative to its consequences showing up in our war against our nature. Such has become an incomprehensible war against our life and ourselves.

Upon reflection it's difficult to see humans avoiding the consequences of wars. In the big one nature is seen to be losing the war with humans, as seen in science, but science says little about what and how we can change the process. An attempt was made to do such in a 1975-77 research project, to be discussed later, where we recommended human change. During the 40 years since that study we have only worked to expand that which must be stopped to survive. It's hard to describe this as anything except "humans are fucked," or

---

[27] In January 1968 I was brought up on charges during combat conditions for refusing an order from my leader. I had been ordered to shoot at women and children fleeing. I responded I preferred to shoot him. From a battlefield prehearing, I was found not guilty and recommended for promotion. The captain was later shot in the back of his head. Humans are funny people.

on a suicide trek. In "The Denial of Death" Ernest Becker described the immortality trek as the essence of evil. For his effort and clarity, he received the 1973 Pulitzer Prize in Nonfiction.

The human dream of continuance for immortality of self or as a member of an immortal species is coming to an end. The problem is how we came to define and thus meet bio-needs and their psycho-wants. From defining the values then the economic processes used to organize work, we destroy the conditions of the context that defines life. Somehow humans have learned to disregard needs for maintaining the quality of context. This may stem from their mental overloads, or as mentioned before seeing how our death is defined at birth.

Strange questions of how nature has been organized continually present challenges to our consciousness. Perhaps they even define our unconsciousness during sleep? Is this what we call life? During our education we come to be told that humans are the crowning achievement in Darwin's hierarchy types. Why then should we tolerate being mortal? In addition, why would we care about our context and its maintenance? Can't nature develop low level species to do such in support of human greatness? Via the development of our science and technology we surely can find doorways into immortality, and negative entropy as will be introduced in what follows. Our literature and books of science are filled with such dreams. But, if we are so great, why should we be lessened by needing to become tolerant of others, and nature?

The essential message in this book is that humans have a fixation on what is immortal, hoping they will find a way to be added to the list, if there are any phenomena outside the entropy process. Wanting to belong to the immortal explains much of what humans dedicate their lives to doing and having. Discovering such seems impossible for life is what sends them towards and sometimes through the doorway of evil. As such they sell their long-term, their soul, for as much short-term gain as they can capture. This is the essence of the Faustian story, his negotiation with, bargaining over and tragedy of life. Such is the context that breeds human warfare with nature (as entropy), others (as a culture of fighting over differences that are not different), and self (in search of a resolution to those self-designed psycho-needs).

Such explains much that is the wrong, and where might we find the right. This helps to explain why humans were drawn to Plato, Confucius, Aristotle, etc. in their quest to make immortality logical. Negotiating with development of technology then pushing the dream to the limits via the industrialization of life illustrates the deeply felt question for immortality from behavior. Thinking about this may well offer the best explanation of why and how humans can be so enamored with artificial intelligence and robots. Such is seen at the societal and personal levels as touchstones of the immortal. It is important therein to ignore the warnings of John Brunner then Stephen Hawking in reminding us that all that is human needs maintenance, including humans. As such they live via the entropic process and thereby are mortal. Robots are as subject to mortality as humans are. To see this is fundamental to resolution of relations to climate change consequence as removal of such consequences is no longer possible. The alternative to such, as the pathway we are on is to accept and pretend to tolerate "Human Beings Being Fucked."

The thesis beneath the work in this book deals with why humans become angry with nature, each other, and themselves via life. Herein the argument is that as humans become more aware of their own mortality and the fragile nature of their life they become upset. If this is untrue then we must find a way to explain why younger children are not upset with nature, each other nor themselves. To examine other thesis please review the Pulitzer Prize winning book *The Denial of Death* by Ernest Becker, 1973. Therein he argued as to how evil in humans was generated in the denying of death as an immortality project. While on a project to explain this in more detail in a follow up work, *Escape From Evil*, 1975 he died. Not a very popular work, it seemed far too clear to want to embrace yet it was basic to my design of the Swedish environmental deterioration project reported herein that described in 1977 how and why humans were creating climate change consequences as an alarming rate. Without the same terminology Becker felt the same in 1974.

At its most elemental level the human organism, like crawling life, has a mouth, digestive tract, and anus, a skin to keep it intact, and appendages with which to acquire food. Existence, for all organismic life, is a constant struggle to feed – a struggle to incorporate whatever other organisms they can fit into their mouths and press down their gullets without choking. Seen in these stark terms, life on this planet is a gory spectacle, a science-fiction nightmare in which digestive tracks fitted with teeth at one end are tearing away at whatever flesh they can reach, and at the other end are piling up the fuming waste excrement as the move along in search of more flesh. I think this is why the...

And this brings us to the unique paradox of the human condition: that man wants to persevere as does any animal or primitive organism; he is driven by the same craving to consume, to convert energy, and to enjoy continued experience. But man is cursed with a burden that no other animal has he is conscious that his own end is inevitable, that his stomach will die.[28]

Humans? They clearly have a problem inherent in their being. One way to access the problem is to decide if it arises from humans as mean or dumb. Wrongdoing is doing what is wrong, but the question is the wrongfulness from a desire to do such, or being so dumb that the good is not accessible.

Meanness is prompted by and arises from the conception of evil. When you feel mean is the order of the day you turn and draw from the well of the evil, which is potentially powerful, maybe even bottomless.

Dumb relates to a lack of intelligence on a subject due to having not researched it, read about it, or considered it. You have not felt a need to do any of that proverbial homework on the subject. This can be seen in a person's driving routine. If they tend to be a rightest they

---

[28] Ernest Becker, *Escape From Evil*, New York: Free Press, 1975. Pp. 2-3.

find it reassuring to simply turn right at each intersection given a choice. If leftist they will always turn left at all choices. Each can then be seen going round and round in circles and being angry each time they meet, often. When they desire to accomplish something else they need to be more flexible, and perhaps even be in the same car.

2. Entropy: The Context of Life

As biological beings we are presented with that biological death certificate as life begins, as mentioned before. What is the meaning of all of this, or is there no meaning to life? How did we get stuck in the context defined and defiled by entropy? Can't we discover and develop a pathway of negative entropy? Einstein and others would mostly say no: Their quotes at entropy.com.

Albert Einstein:

Thermodynamics is the only physical theory of universal content concerning which I am convinced that, within the framework of the applicability of its basic concepts, it will never be overthrown."

Erwin Schrodinger added:

The organism feeds on negative entropy. A living organism feeds upon negative entropy... Thus the device by which an organism maintains itself stationary at a fairly high level of orderliness (= fairly low level of entropy) really consists in continually sucking orderliness from its environment.

To which Aldous Huxley added:

One thinks one's something unique and wonderful at the center of the universe, when in fact one's just a slight inter-ruption in the ongoing march of entropy.

Then, Howard Kunstler Continued:

> Under the current high energy/high entropy regime, sustainable development is a joke. The aggressive incoherence of our common surroundings can be described as entropy made visible. The way we have disposed things on the landscape leads us in the direction of disorder and death. They are categorically evil. These dispositions are destroying our only home-planet and other organisms that share it. They defeat our need to care about where we are and the things in place there. They prompt us to feel that civilization is not worth carrying on. They rob us of our identity and our will to live. These things are not about personal taste or style.

Death certificates should be ignored but more clearly such is seriously beyond human control, or timing. Healthcare of life has grown into an industrial sector, and thus attracts much money, employees many people, and thus has become largely irrelevant to life. Entropy defines its success, not its marketing. As immortality is thus barred from humans they become upset about such and invest negative entropy in subjects such as "life," "cybernetics," "Artificial Intelligence, etc. From an outsider to all of these we thus appear as fucked in all senses of the concept. We thus are thus trapped in a definition of life that places us in a tight spot yet allows for no escape clauses, even by lawyers.

It thus now seems strange to confront criticism of a book title, not its contents describing the end of life from searching for neg-entropy. All this somehow comes to be consistent with the central message of the book. Herein we address the pattern of humans dismissing the long-term then ignoring the cumulative threats of environmental deterioration via human definitions of life's enhancement.

The threats to life were great in 1979, as seen in the study briefly reported herein. Efforts were made to change this, but by 2019 it was clear that the results of the early threats had become ominous. By 2023 we have now passed beyond questioning the 1979 thesis. There are now daily reports on expanding droughts, widening floods, growing heat, and painful deaths. Many purchasing the prior book pointed out they did not plan to read it but loved its title on the bookshelf behind them during their Zoom calls.

By 2022 94% of scientists have come to agree with the thesis found herein, but in more poetic language. The unambiguous title seems consistent with the emerging feeling in the youth seeing their futures affected by failed ideas of prior humans.

> Drastic changes will occur. These will come from attempts at business as unusual as well as that which stimulates it. If the threats from climate change consequences are as harsh as those articulated by Exxon scientists in the 1975-77 research project, then very deep change will occur by and in humans. The danger is that more may be required of humans than what they are capable of. [29] (1977 quotation in the 1979 book introduction.)

Some see no problem in the human future. Via technological development driven by science the challenges will seemingly become resolved or turned into opportunities as they emerge. Editors Rebecca Solnit & Thelma Young illustrate this idea. They ask for optimism in responses to my 2019 book on "Too Early, Too Late, Now what?" with their forthcoming book: "Not Too Late: Changing the Climate Story from Despair to Possibility." Their thesis is consistent with the negative entropy approach mentioned before that has been around for the past two thousand years of human development with emphasis on the past two hundred years of industrial development. We come to justify generation of negative entropy ideas via our position on top of Darwin's hierarchy of being. Standing on such we will surely find ways to avoid the climate change consequences on our horizon that are consistent with entropy processes and speeding

---

[29] David L. Hawk, *Too Early, Too Late, now what?* Thomasville, NC :Brilliant Books, 2022, P. 282

them up. Somehow the credence grows in support of a viewpoint offered in 1969 by Ernest Fisher:

> With increasing momentum, increasingly large masses of human being, goods, inventions, and technical achievements are moving towards a future whose face is veiled and whose body is a chimera, a machine with an archangel's wings, a fantastically rapid alternation of ultra-light and deep, terrible night....
>
> We are lagging behind ourselves. We are unable to catch up with what we have done. We overfeed the sky with the accomplishments of our technology whilst two thousand million people on earth are undernourished. What ought to serve us dominates us. What frees us from effort robs us of our freedom. What the mind devises, power abuses.[30]

My 1979 book, mentioned before, has now been republished four times with different covers, titles, and/or contents. This allowed comparison and discovery of what is most important to those buying books. The content thesis is the same in all five. It looks at the consequences of industrial production, products, and pollution in meeting bio-needs and psycho-wants of humans.

3. Entropy Defines Out Future: Ignore, Deny, Defy

What is this entropy thing? What does it have to do with anything of the lives or humans or processes of nature? As one of the least taught subjects in all universities yet revered laws of science by the most revered scientists it is worth understanding something of entropy and its role in defining the future of human and natural affairs. When I was Prof Eric Trist's teaching/research assistant in 1974/75 I would offer the following story to his MBA classes, to question their myths about the role of their species in the world.

---

[30] Ernst Fischer, *Art Against Ideology*, New York, George Braziller, 1969, p. 37.

This was to reduce their arrogance implicit in their being accepted into a Wharton MBA program. I would begin with the question: "Assuming there is a grand design in nature, what is nature's purpose for humans existing?" My often-used response centered on the concept of entropy. It is generally seen as a confusing concept often remarked as: I first learned of it via a sadly confused instructor in my thermodynamics class at Iowa State University. For him entropy was the concept that he cautioned us to avoid at all costs if we wanted to be successful. To me, it thus became a clear construct in education that clarified much about humans and the universe but requires moving beyond the limits of that Iowa State physics instructor in 1963, the one not wanting to waste his course time on entropy.

For Steven Hawking, the 2nd Law of Thermodynamics was sacrosanct. It was the same for most of the great scientists relative to the fundamental underpinning of entropy in science. The question then becomes: when did humans avoid its inclusion in thinking of economics and laws of nature?

"What must the laws of nature be like so that it is impossible to construct a perpetual motion machine from either the first or the second kind?"[31] This is important to deterioration as most human activities around the ideals of industrialization act as if they are negative entropy. Leading scientists have consistently moved deeper to argue why they agree with Einstein and Hawking as to why entropy is a supreme law of nature and must be factored into humans acts.

"The second law of thermodynamics is, without a doubt, one of the most perfect laws in physics. Any *reproducible* violation of it, however small, would bring the discoverer great riches as well as a trip to Stockholm. The world's energy problems would be solved in one stroke. It is not possible to find any other law (except, perhaps, for super selection rules such as charge conservation) for which a proposed violation would bring more skepticism than this one. Not even Maxwell's laws of electricity or Newton's law of gravitation are so sacrosanct, for each has measurable corrections coming from quantum effects or general relativity. The law has caught the attention of poets

[31] Klein, Martin, *Science*, Vol. 157, 509, 1967

and philosophers and has been called the greatest scientific achievement of the nineteenth century. Engels disliked it, for it supported
opposition to Dialectical Materialism, while Pope Pius XII regarded
it as proving the existence of a higher being."[32]

If someone approaches you declaring they discovered "neg-entropy" beware. On the one hand they probably do not understand
entropy. On the other hand they may indeed know its definition but
selling a bowl of phony happiness wrapped in falsehood to invite you
into the world of the immoral via knowing of entropy yet moving
into making and marketing of products as neg-entropy. In the class
in question I would go further to describe how much of what is
designed, produced, and sold in an industrial-based society focuses
on, not just the possibility of neg-entropy, but its products being
widely available. None-the-less, the universe remains subject to the
entropy law, and it is not to be defied by economic mythologies.

> "The law that entropy always increases holds, I think, the
> supreme position among the laws of Nature. If someone
> points out to you that your pet theory of the universe is in
> disagreement with Maxwell's equations — then so much
> the worse for Maxwell's equations. If it is found to be con-
> tradicted by observation — well, these experimentalists do
> bungle things sometimes. But if your theory is found to be
> against the second law of thermodynamics, I can give you
> no hope; there is nothing for it but to collapse in deepest
> humiliation."[33]

Back to the story I outlined in a previous section that stimulates
the above definitions and concerns: Why did nature invent humans?
Thousands of years ago nature encountered a violation of her entropy
law in a pocket of neg-entropy in the earth. It was a clear violation of
her supreme rule. She was unsure how to clean up the mess resulting

---

[32] Bazarov, Ivan P., *"Thermodynamics,"* 1964
[33] Sir Arthur Stanley Eddington, *The Nature of the Physical World* (1915), chapter 4

from the violation. A euphemistic means to understand entropy is seen in repeated meetings with it, prior to being trapped. I presented this to that professor in my first Physics class at ISU in 1963. Yes, he failed me. He told me I was fucked. He was right.

Encounter: *There is a game.*

First Law: You can't win.

Second Law: You must lose.

Third Law: You can't quit.

The problem was that much petroleum from dinosaur remains came to be entrapped deep underground, and via entropy it could not be entropic dissipation via doing work arriving at cold disorder via time. That storehouse of potential to do work that was fixed in time was in violation of entropy, the 2nd Law of Thermodynamics. What was nature to do to resolve this contradiction to her fundamental law? She arrived at the idea of inventing a being that would go and release all that buried neg-entropy so a natural order could arrive at. Within about 100,000, a very short time, she became pleased with her result – much of the petroleum was being released into the air. This being that solved her problem came to be called humans. She then only needed to await the distribution of petroleum into the air then she would get rid of these humans.

Students listening to this never seemed to laugh. This simple-minded story reveals much in our world, including the problem of humans relating to nature. Yes, many prefer the explanation in the fourth encounter above, "You can't quit."

The values behind the current state of humankind and its relations to the environment are consistent with Newton's dream of industrialization based on reason. The concern behind this document is closer to Einstein's thinking and concerns about what men should and shouldn't do. This concern is herein centered on continuation of business as seen in business as usual. As such it is akin to the values behind a Native American proverb: "We don't inherit the earth from our ancestors, we borrow it from our children."

Such a value, or the lack thereof, seems central to what humans do and thus crucial to the problems articulated herein. For some reason(s) contemporary human's give emphasis to ownership of property to define their status, then move forward to borrow against the future of that property and those who will depend on it. The most we humans can think of is to take the property, then borrow against its image based on past value to take over control of neighboring properties to demonstrate future wealth that isn't, all the while getting others to use it as it deteriorates. Clearly this leads to problems that now begin to be seen in small publications like the "Tragedy of the Commons."[34] Concern is now in seeing a general deterioration of land, water, and air by the many for purposes of the few but the problem remains.

The deterioration becomes more serious with time leading to life-threatening conditions on the planet as initiated by human acts. Humans have come to ignore or have ignorance of the consequences of their actions, actions derived from an endemic desire for greater and higher results in ever shorter terms. The two-year Stockholm research project was conducted into this concern then sought two ways to regulate it. The project went well beyond studies of the effectiveness of pieces of regulation to examine the chances for success of analytic (short term) responses to systemic (longer-term consequential) difficulties. The results from the two years of work were clarifying yet troubling. This document attempts to present and explain these results.

The research was set up to examine the role of relationships in leading to long-term consequences of human acts. The relationships were between humans, between humans and nature, then between humans and their images of their selves. All the relations were analyzed with a clearly rational emphasis on cause-effect understanding of parts. This non-systemic approach was taken to help understand the mentality behind the actions, not the systemic consequences of those actions. That was examined later. The non-systemic was found to be based in a desire for stability via the values of changelessness. An alternative value set emerged from participants at the edge of operations; those who lived in a world of change. As a sign of there

---

[34] "Tragedy of the Commons, *Science*, 1965

being a better way towards problem resolution the results of the study point to the clarity of views coming from the edges; those who embraced change and practiced fluid management of connections, not parts. Those bound by analysis could only see parts, not connections. Those thinking systemically came to mostly see connections while overlooking behavior of parts. As such, the project focus became critical of standard economic thinking, acting and fixing. The project did examine how humans arrive at valuations; especially what and how they arrive at value of life?

Humans seem to be developing what is herein called the *human project*. In its essence, the current stage of development is seen to be based in Newtonian-directed industrialization values. These seek the mechanical rationality that can be seen in emphasizing causal results from backward analysis of effects. Herein this is seen as 1-dimensional greed as managed by 2-dimensional regulation based on paper. Ostensibly, the purpose of the human project is to supply human needs with reduced human work all while encouraging humans to seek fulfillment in life through inventing and seeking material wants.

Meanwhile, humans tend to not notice, or not care, about the peripheral costs in the ever-expanding human project's environmental deterioration from one–dimensional thinking as seen in three-dimensional danger to life. This, added to the irreversible nature of natural entropic deterioration, pose serious problems for systems of living order. Early responses to this, by those humans who notice something amiss, is, once again, 1-dimensional ideas set out on 2-dimensional paper to manage the complexities of 3-dimensional deterioration. Those who seem to most understand the situation see all this as *a band aid awaiting surgery.*

The research was set up to improve understanding of the current situation, then to propose ideas for changing human values about human relations to their environment and the entities occupying it. Research results raised questions about control over emerging conditions, or lack of any control. Evidence suggested that humans lack control over themselves thus how can they hope to control the consequences of environmental conditions they have changed? That became the research question after the research results were written up. Many reviewing the results responded that "tougher regulations and enforcement" were needed. A few argued that we need to await further expansion of current rude experiences from a deteriorating environment, to mobilize political action. Via this pain from "effects," humans would more efficiently work to identify and control the "causes." Then, the effects would be erased and the negative consequences to the planet would be avoided. In this way industrial production pollution and further pollution from the use of industrial products would be taken care of. As such the human project could continue. The history of philosophy, science and humanism illustrates that this myth was not to be realized. Neg-entropy would not be discovered and realized.

The research data showed why this myth could not happen. Thus, significant changes to the human project and the values sponsoring it are needed. The roles of the analytic (i.e., the rational) and systemic (i.e., the non-rational) must be changed, perhaps even reversed. Without such this phenomenon called the human project will become buried by other forces.

There were two major research concerns. 1) The first was with the limits in knowledge of environmental deterioration in three dimensions, and the consequences of this in the fourth dimension. Hundreds of industry and university researchers in many countries pointed to the data for this in the project. 2) The second, and perhaps more serious, concern was seen in seriously humorous reliance on one-dimensional thinking to govern two-dimensional regulatory governance. This did not appreciate, nor have any chance to manage, the highly systemic domain of 4-dimensional consequences. It even failed to manage deterioration of the third dimension. Hundreds of governmental and legal researchers in several countries helped describe this dilemma for the human project.

The level of understanding in both problem domains seemed locked into the limitations of traditions in their respective domains. Both seemed to come from Paramedian and Platonic arguments for reality as changelessness. As they said, if it changes it is no more, thus why worry about it? It's like the weather. As such, humans continue to be troubled in conceiving of Socratic, Heraclitan worlds ruled by ideas of nature and natural change. The world of the artificial is paramount to the human project, especially artificial stability.

The science limitation comes from the reductionistic tradition set by Newtonian dissection and analytic methods to seek cause-effect two-dimensional relationships. In so thinking humans avoid thinking of death and related timetable dilemmas. These are of the four-dimensional effects of nature that lie beyond human powers or understanding. Concern for this came to be one of many shortcomings showing up in the research. One researcher pointed out how she felt trapped in the limits of her university education where she went to learn about nature but was instead taught cause-effect thinking was fundamental to knowledge. In this way she jokingly pointed out that what she learned from the fox chasing the rabbit allowed her to know that the rabbit was perhaps the cause of the fox. Prior to graduation she was encouraged to move to the edges of reality and appreciate, or even understand, the systemic phenomena operating there, e.g., nature.

Limitations beyond the simple-minded analytics were found in the second area, the regulatory. Regulation approaches were set up to approximate changelessness in a situation. In this way those having control over the situation could remain in control. The research evidence showed how the values of stability via changelessness were endemic to management of industrialization. The "externalities" of avoiding change were seen in the same dim light. Widely advertised domains of Platonic truth and justice, as the espoused bedrock of regulation, were seldom noted or noticed after graduation from law school. The two soon joined the trash pile containing any ideas of ethics. Ethics were quickly set aside in college instruction. Students learned that ethics and the law were two very different domains, and they should avoid the confusion of ethics and concentrate on warm certainty in the law as written. Ideas of including a larger setting in a more systemic manner, such as including a wider social group as the problem, were simply side-stepped. More radical ideas such as including laws of nature in laws of man, or even including the natural environment in environmental laws, as the location of the problematique, were avoided.

Throughout the study it appeared that regulation was to maintain the operations of "business as usual." The often-used metaphor by those who knew was we need regulation to "keep the lid on things" until we figure out what is going on and what to do. To accommodate all these contradictions, regulation thus needed to absorb much ambiguity. This was specifically done via developing and relying on legalism as communication to those that expected more. Users and religious adherents of the American approach to the law, i.e., words on paper, and the essential basis to regulation, argued how even if laws are not written clearly they did allow a bit of room for movement, i.e., essential deceit needed in and out of regulator's offices and courtrooms. To non-lawyers this tactic becomes obvious with time. Non-lawyers would easily see that the language of law, as "legalize," was essential to hide what lawyers fail to know and cannot express even in two dimensions. Knowing this allows you to see how one-dimensional enforcement of laws is clear, then clearly counter-productive.

Problems with drawing up laws and enforcing them to solve societal problems was seen in capital crime and drug usage expansions attempted during the nineteen-sixties. The same limitations are now becoming noticeable in the environmental legislation of the late sixties and early seventies. Not only is ambiguity not to be avoided in the US approach to writing laws; it is essential to accommodate an almost complete lack of knowledge about a systemically connected terrain.

Thus, both science and regulation are trapped in the limitations of what Gregory Bateson called "unaided rationality." Both had a reliance on concepts like logic and accepted the serious limitations that resulted from using them to attempt management of a systemic nature. To regain a place in the natural world, before it is too late, we must give up our simplistic, quantitative science….and learn, as Bateson suggests, "to think like Nature thinks…"[35] Or, to be clearer about the everyday limitations on human thinking seen in unques-

---

[35] *Mind and Nature*, Bateson, Gregory, Bantam Books: Toronto, 1978, inside cover

tioned frameworks of thought we need only recall the definition of logic presented near the beginning of this book.

Moving to the broader context of limitations seen in social regulation, as we now practice it, we need only look at the extensive use of ambiguously drawn and interpreted regulations. One hint of how bad this is can be seen in reliance on 125 plus word sentences, where the writing seems to not know why they enter and certainly have no idea of how to exit. Following are guidelines to "help" those preparing Environmental Impact Statements to send to court and other places:

> "Agency procedures shall also specifically include provision for public hearings on major actions with environmental impact, whenever appropriate, and for providing the public with relevant information, including information on alternative courses of action in deciding whether a public hearing is appropriate, and agency should consider: (1) the magnitude of the proposal in terms of economic cost, the geographical area involved, and the uniqueness or size of commitment of the resources involved...[36]

The above 70-word introduction to the sentence does continue for another 90 words. Therein a humorously strong statement, that this law: "...shall also specifically include provision....", is soon followed by a noteworthy qualifier of: ".... whenever appropriate...." Seeming clarity, using ambiguous sentence structure to wrap around specific double-talk is seen throughout thousands of pages in this and related environmental laws and rules of enforcement.

When the research study results were presented to OECD by Sweden's Government, they used it to denote the "American approach to regulation." The Swedish alternative came from the quotation of the Swedish Minister of Environment: "We Swedes are, it seems, unusual in that we believe the first stage to get citizens to obey a law

---

[36] *Federal Register*, US Government, Vol. 38, No. 147 – Wednesday, August 1, 1973m o, 20, 553.

is to understand it." The US Head of EPA at the time, wrote me a letter of some hostility about this "nasty" comment. Others found the comment informative then insightful.

The study began in 1975 with direct knowledge of wholly ineffective results from 1969 legislation. Clearly, another approach was needed to begin management of harmful human actions on the natural environment, or, to at least prepare for consequences of continuance and mismanagement. Conclusions pointed to some hope in development of the positive nature of environmental appreciation for improving human-nature relations. The common practice in 1975 was based on legalistic punishment for being caught doing what a law deemed as wrong. The first approach was to encourage a search for better understanding and responses to problems in human relations and was called "business as unusual." The second approach was seen to be sidestepping of societal restrictions that were not well understood nor open to legalistic practice but came to encourage more "business as unusual."

Specific difficulties are depicted in some detail in the reporting of the research behind this document as seen in "Environment Protection: Analytic Solutions in Search of Synthetic Problems," 1977. This was published by the Institute of International Business, Stockholm School of Economics and presented by Sweden to OECD in raising questions about the legalistic emphasis in the US approach to environmental concern.

Leadership was found to be a key control factor in the study, especially with those given overriding authority to resolve or create problems. The study found that too much leadership was centered on those with a very limited education in the law as written by humans, i.e., lawyers, and/or in those trained to be on top a hierarchy as nurtured in business school education. On the other hand, those in direct supervision of production and governmental oversight were granted little authority yet illustrated a very different sense of environmental problems. Many impediments to business as unusual were set up in corporate headquarters or central government offices. This created dilemmas in narrowly conceived designs of production processes followed by similar regulatory means to control the negative consequences of it all.

Each model of design of course finds dilemmas but fixating then freezing a single model tends to worsen things as it is deterred from adaptation at the edges. There was much humor in the obvious contradictions revealed in the research, but the cumulative results were of course not funny. This was especially clear in US examples where there was the greatest fixation on one right way. In one state they encountered a problem with what to do with toxic waste. The lawyers involved had no idea of what to do so they passed legislation that denied its existence. Within two years it had to be rescinded. In another state it was discovered that all wells in a region contained dangerous to life chemical. The seemingly irresolvable problem was dealt with via cutting off future funds to measure water quality.

VII

EFFECTS FROM PRIOR EFFECTS, NOT FROM FUTURE CAUSES

Humans, particularly those schooled in Plato/Aristotle thinking about what is going on and to go on, go for the simple. Even where it is wrong, which it often is, they stick with the simple. When you ask for their definition of "simple" they end up talking via complicated terms of bad definitions. Somehow when humans need to take shelter they do so under the term complex. When they want to be well regarded they pose theories for management of complexity. Why they want to go for the simple minded while embracing the term complex for the results not working is a humanistic mystery. Listen carefully and you should be able to see examples of this from your friends and family. Of course dealing with a managerial boss is simpler. He tells you want he wants, and you think "fucking idiot" as you sort of listen, gently smile and nod to show agreement. The same pattern shows up in confronting the law and those lawyers, judges and policemen that try to enforce such, except, depending on how much pay they expect, they too can take you to the complex. Marital relations are somewhat similar.

The importance of seeing the common use, i.e., misuse, of simple and complex carries over into the extensive use of cause-effect thinking and speaking in schools, science, job, home, and community, which begins to reveal the trouble humans are in and why. Let's

101

look closer at what is known as "cause-effect" thinking, with emphasis on its mentor, Aristotle.

We are told that "cause" states the "why" of something happening. We are then told that "effect" directs us to a "resulting outcome." When I once argued with county officials for wanting to cut down a bird-filled tree near a stream on my fathers farm. I said the effect would be the loss of homes for hundreds of birds and they would be the cause. They argued that with the tree gone the stream would run much faster and get the water to the river more efficiently, an effect sorely needed. I countered with the rapidly running water would also take the underlying soil along to the river (the Mississippi). In effect they then told me I was dumb with the effect being I told them to "fuck off." The effect of that was they wanted to charge me for threatening them as the cause of what they would then do. I wrote an article in the local paper about the sweet, happy birds and how we should slow water run-off, not speed it up, thus saving soil. The effect of that was the citizens argued for firing the county workers for being so dumb and mean. The tree remained.

Most of us end up investing our lives in such "negotiations" with most of it being based on knowledge of nothing and the driving force being to win the argument no matter how wrong it and its consequences might be. This explains much of the teaching of Russell Ackoff at the Wharton School to MBA students. He, and his students, really enjoyed him making fun of what were accepted as fundamental of good management. The first and most basic of these was the idea of Greeks as interpreted by Adam Smith and others of economic success being measured via the industrial as continual improvement of productivity. As such the cause of a good economy was assumed to be improved efficiency, even if it was a better job in doing the wrong thing.

Ackoff would instead argue that the students once they were in jobs was to find and do the right thing, even if it was done inefficiently. He thus argued for continual change in improving what was being done more than in doing it better. His examples of his work as senior advisor to many of the major US companies were spellbinding. As the founder of the discipline and mathematics of Operations

Research he gave emphasis to learning of change based on improvement of end states, not processes. When OR turned against his model he left and want into systems thinking and said, "The future of OR is in its past, and they missed it."

As you can imagine, he was one of my favorite teachers, even when he was wrong, as we all are on occasion. He and I argued often about many fun things. His emphasis in moving to systems approaches to seeing problems was very helpful to me, but he did retain aspects of cause-effect thinking to dissect such problems. Herein I go a step further to abandon the cause-effect model of Aristotle, who argued for humans moving into a causal investigation of the world.

Prior to Aristotle we see in Plato's *Phaedo* that "inquiry into nature" is a search for "the causes of each thing; why each thing comes into existence, why it goes out of existence, why it exists" (96 a 6-10) As such a search for causes was to answer all questions of "why?". Aristotle continued Plato's tradition but criticized that Plato and all before him had no clear distinctions and clarity with cause-effect. In his *Metaphysics* Aristotle commented that they were like boxers lacking boxing technique: while sometimes they can throw a nice punch, any punch that lands is only a lucky one (Aristotle, Metaphysics, I4, 985 a 10-19).

The essence of Aristotle's "definition" of "causes" seems complex. Probably it is, as most definitions tend to be. He posed there to be four kinds of causes. They are:

1. "The material cause of that which is given in reply to the question "What it made out of?" What is singled out in the answer need not be material objects such as bricks, stones, or planks. By Aristotle's lights, A and B are the material cause of syllable BA.
2. The formal cause or that which is given I reply to the question "What is it?". What is singled out in the answer is the essence of the what-it-is-to-be something.
3. The efficient cause or that which is given I reply to the question "Where does change (or motion) come from?".

What is singled out in the answer is the whence of change (or motion).

4. The final cause is that which is given in reply to the question: "What is its good?". What is singled out in the answer is that for the sake of which something is done or takes place." [37]

If you want to go beyond the limits of Aristotle you might look at The Paradox of Cause to begin to see the serious limits of causal thinking and the need to drop such or redefine its operations. As its author says:

> The expulsion of mind and purpose from the domain of nature offers no novelty in the history of thought. But in our own day, determinism and mechanism are no longer esoteric beliefs but generally accepted axioms. To be sure, one often encounters pious affirmations of faith in some supernatural agency, in the soul, or in immortality; but such faith has degenerated into a vague hope, into an attractive but hardly defensible aspiration. Nowadays one needs to apologize for teleology, whereas mechanism no longer labors under the burden of proof. Even psychology openly boasts of its emancipation from the ghost-soul and complacently displays its wares in terms of stimulus-response events…Apparently we cannot rest in meaningless and lawless variety. [38]

We can also go to that very easy to follow dictionary that clarifies much in complex life:

> "Effect, n. The second of two phenomena which always occur together in the same order. The first, called a Cause,

---

[37] *Stanford Encyclopedia of Philosophy*, "Aristotle on Causality," March 7, 2023.

[38] John William Miller, *The Paradox of Cause*, New York: W.W. Norton & Co., 1978, p. 11.

is said to generate the other – which is no more sensible than it would be for one who has never seen a dog except in pursuit of a rabbit to declare the rabbit the cause of the dog." (Devils Dictionary, New York: Hill and Wang, 1881.)

Perhaps it's time to go easy on cause-effect logic at the center of our thinking when humans bother to even think. From my research in the seventies I could show that use of cause-effect logic in factories and regulatory agencies was a major method for control, then a major "cause" of why the situation was even more out of control. Participants question, such as when Senator Muskie wanted to know my alternative, was "What would you recommend?"

From looking at the data collected from factories on failures to control pollution and then asking where we were going as humans if this continues I began to talk about a different kind of systems approach to capture the complexity that each argument arrived at yet let the process be easily understandable. That was when I began to talk about noticeable effects in need of management tended to come from other effects sort of hidden, or attempted to be hidden, in the past. As such attempts to manage those effects would lead to more effects.

My Prime example was how air and water quality regulations were used to govern pollution from a pulp and paper factory in Florida. EPA lauded it as the cleanest paper factory in the nation. Plant managers thought the award was undeserved as the pollution was not eliminated, only buried in the back of the site where eventually they knew it would leak into ground water. None-the-less it did not go directly into the air as before. They agreed with my changing to think of effects of effects model but asked me to not let EPA management know about their feelings.

We now arrive in a situation well beyond the consequences of air, water, and solid waste pollution of humans. Climate Change Consequences do not fit into that Aristotelian model. The process leading to such is much more systemic and thus easier to see if you forget the rewards you are used to getting from discovering causes of effects.

When you have time think about the use of the Aristotle model of cause-effect to explain inflation. We listen to arguments from bankers and former bankers that attempt to regulate money flows that its due to money supply, interest rates, and factors of economic stimulation from government. When you get a change for a bit of thought of how climate change relates to inflation of food and housing prices please forget the discussions you hear on TV and in classrooms. Instead step back and see the Second Law of Thermodynamics, the Entropy Law, as the effect of permanent inflationary effects. Such began with time and will continue after time is gone. Such also suggests a very different approach to management of the consequences of inflation via entropy. You can also use the effect of Covid from prior effects of human-nature relations and distant effects of expanded the disease base bit global warming.

No, I'm not saying cause-effect thinking "causes" climate change, but it sure does not encourage thinking of it in a way to avoid it or manage it. Sorry.

1. Change as Entropic Reality: Changelessness as False Immortality

Herein we rely on effects of effects thinking to make sense of the entropic process, the basis for natural change, as well as the creator of the notion of time. Life is herein seen as change in nature, not artificially fixation locked into a cube for retaining changelessness. Humans have trouble with this. Most lock their dreams into changelessness. My concern is with how this keeps humans from seeing the process and effects of climate change, and its consequences. They prefer to roll around in a dream of non-existence captured in a fixed definition of everyday existence. As such humans place much value on the thinking of life as changelessness as articulated by Parmenides, born about 515 BCE. He defined how changelessness is reality. Socrates argued the opposite until 399 BCE but was then executed. As such we see that a majority of humans then and now prefer the

Parmenidean argument of life as changeless. In his single publication of his poem of life he states:

> "What Is has some type of timeless existence....What Is does not come to be more by passing away..." (Parmenidean Metaphysical Poem on Life, Fr. 8.5-6a)

If something changes than by Parmenidean logic it isn't. Herein it is argued that those seeing no problem from and in climate change are akin to the Parmenidean School of Philosophy. On the other hand the philosophical school of his opponent, Heraclitus, is very consistent with the emergence of climate change and its consequences for life. Heraclitus saw our world divided into true and false, one and many, and being and non-being. Heraclitus endorsed, even embraced the idea of life as paradoxical things, and that methods of humans are essentially impossible. For Heraclitus if something does not change it is the essence of dead, as it is without life and the basis of life is change.

As such, in what follows the idea of C^3 = *Climate Change Consequences* is crucial to what we might see as truth about Parmenidean extreme valuation in an idea of Changelessness. It seems the same for those that devalue climate change, green paint our vision over its evidence, and advise us to not worry, as "the weather is always changing, so what?"

2. Changelessness, A Religion

Permanence embraced in constancy seems to be a basic value from the industrial age. Constancy is artificial but is often used in management under conditions of rapid change from visions of technological potential. Changelessness values of humans assume great responsibility for problems in how humans deal with the natural context in that nature is defined by change. This is how humans came to define their war with the natural.

The cube in 3 Dimensions provides us with a fundamental metaphor: The human existence via the brain, not the mind, is best seen as a cube. This offers us a 3-D cube that offers and contains a calm, simple situation that symbolizing continuity, stability, and permanence, all realized via geometric perfection. The cube thus becomes the mathematical representation of non-change as a final stage of immobility. The cube represents our finding, or needing to find, a human truth looking the same from all perspectives.

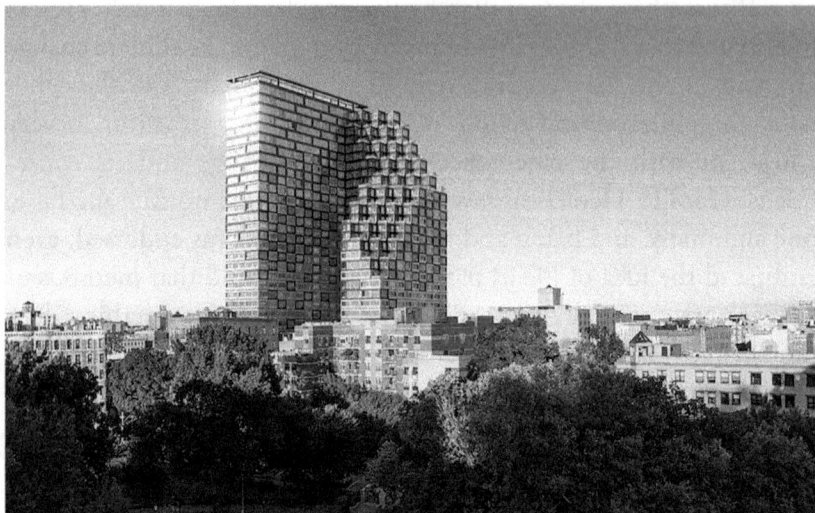

Matt Buchanan, "Boxed in New York City," AWL Network, 2015

It represents control via the world of the artificial squaring of the more natural world seen in the circle. It is the metaphorical box humans tend to sleep, eat, and work within although perhaps the basis for many mental problems to follow. The cube represents the human earth: a square plus four elements in three dimensions. It has frequently been used to form allegories of solidity and the persistence of virtues, hence often related to thrones, chariots, limousines, etc. It thus became and remains the basis for housing humans and their various activities to carry out and maintain life. We might best call it *"life in the box."*

The ocean will rise an estimated 1.6 feet if the vast Thwaites Glacier melts. That melting could start a negative feedback loop that will destabilize more glaciers and raise the waters *almost 10 feet more*.

It's no wonder they nicknamed it the Doomsday Glacier! All the beaches we know in the United States will be toast. Miami will be destroyed. Many South Pacific Islands will be gone. The shape of the world as we now know it will be altered for good.

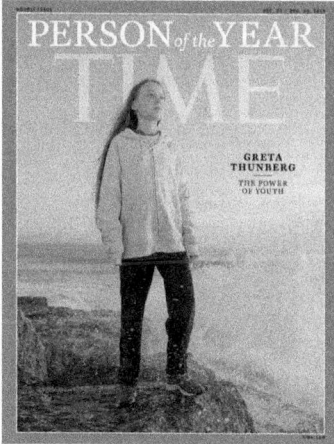

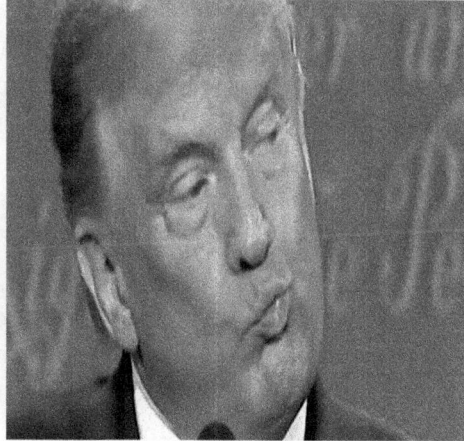

Two Souls: One an arrogant, immature human having little to no knowledge and solely speaks from love of self, not context. The other is Greta Thunberg who talks of change.

Why do we attract the leadership we deserve as seen in our behavior? Is there a God to protect us from our broken souls? Perhaps not....

3. Cracks Let the Light In

Ring the bell which still can ring,
Forget your perfect offering,
There is a crack, a crack, in everything,
That's how the light gets in.
(Leonard Cohen, *Anthem*, 1992)

Cohen describes the situation poetically. Plato, in his Allegory of the Cave, goes deeper into the philosophical aspect and articulates that eternal need of light against dark in life as a context of life. Plato's underground cave keeps out the sunlight of natural life. Therein only the artificial version exist as managed by information from a fire run by select humans with signals in two dimensions on a ceiling.

These pages offer sample situations from my life. Each involves the development of a small crack allowing light into the proverbial Platonic Cave. This is in the nature of Leonard Cohen on larger problems into the darkness of human behavior and the settings associated with such. Let us hope they are unusual. If they are typical or even frequent, then humans are on the wrong side of the contradiction we call life. Conclusion: Humans must learn about Change outside the box where the box is similar to Plato's Cave where humans only experience 2D reality as shadows on the ceiling of the cave from the fire below, similar to humans looking at their TVs and Smartphone screens.

The notion of there being crackage in human results is like that metaphorical hole through which some humans escape from the cruel darkness of Plato's Allegory of the Cave. Elsewhere I argue for the importance of accepting there will be cracks on all that humans attempt to use or create.

To pretend a nonexistence of cracks is similar to holding a belief in human power over cosmic entropy, i.e., immortality in who they are, and thus whatever they do. To the objections of many I call such negative entropy. If you would like a test taste of why 90% of being human is to see negative entropy in what they believe and do. You can quickly get a glimpse of this in looking at any advertising, commercial or billboard inviting you to join infinity. You should note that its qualities are non-natural as in humanly artificial.[39]

Via the cosmic and planetary sciences, we begin to see the need for human concern for what might come to be called crackage management; the management of the effects of prior endeavors thought to be effective in support of some definition of purpose. For humans these are their responses to the search for support of bio-needs and psycho-wants.

---

[39] David Hawk, Annaleena Parhankangas, "Systems Cracks are Where the Light Gets In: Models and Measures of Service In the Benefits of Context," Systems Science in Service to Humanity, *Proceedings of the International Society for the Systems Sciences*, Pacific Grove, Ca. 2001.

Looking through the activity trail of my life I see where it was greatly influenced for concern for "cracks" in what others saw to be their fulfilling worthy objectives. I came to feel their desires, plans and actions were based on false optimism for good, that I will later call negative entropy, or a genuine need to participate in the negative end of entropy. I felt a need to question both but was never sure why. Perhaps I was uninformed, misinformed or simply silly? Perhaps I was being managed by religious feelings, although no religion ever wanted me as part of their form or spuing their content.

A fundamental problem exists in responding to the climate change issue, as seen in humans not responding to what they see, feel, and are very concerned with. They are used to the tradition of problem solving, seeing the problem, find the cause, thus solved.

Much of what humans have come to see as knowledge has emerged from what is known as "cause-effect" thinking. They see or feel an effect then set out to see and even understand its cause. Ultimately, they dream of controlling the effect in this way towards creating more of what they like and less of what is not liked. The word cause has a legal origin. It was derived as a legal term by Greeks and Romans considering actions they did not appreciate in others and thus sought legal remedies in those causing them. In this way they felt they could improve society and its occupants. Eventually humans expanded this into non-human realms of life where a cause could be something present, or something absent, but was indeed something. Much of the history and shortcomings of this approach can be read in the book edited by Daniel Lerner of 1965: Cause and Effect.

4. Seeing The Abyss: "We Are Fucked."

If you become upset with the book's title and these few comments about the agenda of the book, I recommend you move on. When the book was first published Amazon would not allow it to be in their books section. It was placed in candles. I complemented their management for being very insightful for such by pointing out that when customers open the book and became angry they could turn to their candle and burn the damned thing thus showing their role in the unending search for misplaced optimism. When I complemented them on this insightfulness towards making the consumer happy they then moved the book to T-shirts with "bad" words on them. The genius of our marketing systems is amazing. Where will it end? The current attitude towards marketing began in the 1920's via getting females to begin smoking.

For some reason humans want *having, not creating*. As such they behave as *bankers of the artificial, not participants in creating the artificial from the natural*. The mentality is to guard and account what is owned while they become angry watching such be dissipated by entropy, the supreme law of the universe. As they watch and count humans also find they are subject to the death sentence dealt by entropy processes.

To reinforce such reasoning, the reasons of the artificial, they organize education of the youth via skill in memorization of answers, not asking of questions. While being a Research Assistant at the Wharton School, U of Penn, in 1974, I suggested there was a somewhat urgent need to change much of what humans think they know and attempt to do. This arose from my time invested in farming, schooling, fighting in warfare, watching leadership, attending funerals, and seeing nature die off. Just prior to my RA work I had been a project manager for the company of Brown and Goldfarb on a Florida development. I had designed a plan to help 10,000 residents to live in an area with minimal disturbance to the natural swamps and forests. It won praises for seeming to be a new way to build and then was widely approved by local, state, and federal officials. When presented to the development CEO he threw the papers in the trash and smiled as he commented: "Now it's time to get to work and level that terrain." I responded to him that the alligators would enjoy eating him, and his customers.

Back in Philadelphia I was fired by a newly hired MBA graduate "office manager." She thought my behavior was disgusting but claimed I was fired for an earlier event where I showed general disrespect for authority. The week before she had made a long presentation on filling in forms to document 15-minute project work investments. At the end I raised my hand and asked "Where is the category for filling out the form, as such could take more than 15 minutes? She left the room and demanded that Hawk be fired if they needed her skills and talent. She stayed away until I returned from Florida and was then fired. The stated reason was I had failed to show proper respect to authority in the workplace. She later revealed that she was most upset by how I had treated an important client, calling him allegator food? Her MBA training found that unacceptable. The developer was simply fighting for human dignity in its fight with nature to make things better. I left the job pointing out that much of that development would be blown away by storms or underwater by 2050. Those who insisted on human occupation of Florida could make caves to protect against hurricanes then learn to swim in them all day and night. From that they could learn to renegotiate existence with nature. I did not see a desirable future for an undesirable species.

Thereafter I began to notice hope in children under five asking largely ignored questions about their being told to acclimate to their cultures and societal values. From seeing the natural context in some troubles they were asking why is culture more important than a tree? I also noted how they gradually stopped asking questions that mattered, as learned they should prepare for a future where they could become omnipresent. They learned to replace questions of where we are going to concentrating on where are the happiness stores? Humans seemed to be greatly blesses with life yet often acted out of meanness about such going away in a guaranteed death. While driving around in search of meaning I would ask why am I driving around? The previous year I had composed a thesis for an angry faculty on "The Communication Alternative: From Pushing Concrete to Exchanging Ideas."

That thesis felt there to be hope in replacing cars with electronics to related to others then relying on biology to understand nature as a meaningful context, not a subservient storehouse of raw materials. With a touch of humor, I suggested humans should restrain their interactions to electronic messaging then reserve walks in nature for special occasions. I suggested with a smile that there would be fewer divorces and wars if people didn't meet. By 2010 I found out how wrong I had been. Actual meetings were not the problem. It was much deeper and wider than physical meetings.

My associates sort of agreed but said their jobs required "getting along." I guess that meant something between praising the wrong to tolerating the obvious shit in models they were required to respect further up the hierarchy. I recommended dumping the hierarchy, but that was said to be beyond dangerous. They pointed to the Herbert Simon wisdom that a hierarchy is fundamental to knowledge, for which he received a Nobel Prize. He said hierarchy is the most essential aspect of human's knowing and must be retained. In a later lecture to an audience which Simon was in I went on to argue why hierarchy was essential to the failure of humans.

My Wharton colleagues wouldn't touch dumping hierarchy but did discuss changes to 1) models of business (forgetting Harvard's strategic thinking as it was and is deceit), 2) financial measurements of business success (moving away from short-term gain as finance onto longer term thinking via morality), 3) hatred of nature, each other, and selves (I suggested to them that love of such may prove to be essential to a meaningful life). They discussed such but I attempted to practice the three. Thus, I was fired by many places that I had never applied to work at but had been recruited to be associated with. Those three non-hierarchical subjects were seen as important with time but lacking critic of hierarchy and leadership they didn't improve.

I offer this book to my Republican friends as advice for when they are fucked from being out all night in search of suitable sex partners, but failing in such they seek books that must be fondled prior to their burning them. The top of this list are mates that ignore them and books they are incapable of reading based on their early years in school. They then moved down to words from others and book covers that generate the anger that can mask disappointment and rejection from others and books. What they can have sex with or comprehend via reading should clearly be burned. Such rises their symbols of readiness to be important.

Failing in all such explanations for defeat they can turn to their metaphysical inspiration found in their easy-to-read pocketbooks: *Mein Kampf* or *The Art of the Deal* (Steal).

5. Writing About Humans As Fucked

Book (5) *Sorry, Humans are Fucked*, is a less optimistic title of (4) *Human Nature and the Potential in Nurture* by Writer's Branding. Previously there were two versions of *Too Early, Too Late, Now what?* (3) (2), by Brilliant Books and Author House. Both used the same title but different cover images. One was mostly black with a small setting sun in the west. The other was a blue sunshine arising from the remains of California fires. All four appeared 40 years after the original book (1) *Regulation of Environmental Deterioration* as Published by the Wharton School, University of Pennsylvania. It was published by fellow students motivated from an argument with Wharton's Dean about the perspective on nature of most courses being taught in business schools in America.

Book (6) Short-term Gain, Long-term Pain, continues the theme by confronting the "now what" aspect of books (2) and (3). It is mostly sold to universities in Europe for courses in management.

The 1979 book published a 1977 dissertation on dire results as written up in final reports from a 1975-77 research project. Based at the Stockholm School of Economics it outlined the need for humans to redesign business as usual. Environmental pollution was expanding around the earth at an expanding rate. This came from human activities that were expanding and forecast to be dangerous to life forms by 2000. Such would then become deadly by 2050 and devastating by 2100. Results were from 20 companies as identified in the prior section of this book where they were making products and processes which had production facilities in six countries. With this we could compare to see what means were most effective to regulate unwanted aspects of industry.

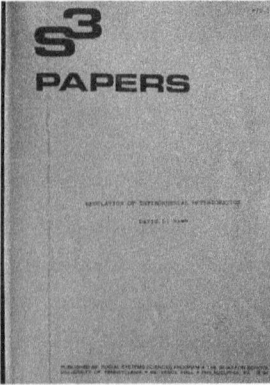
1.

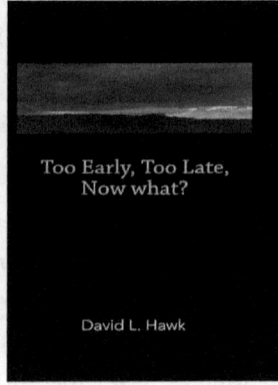
2.

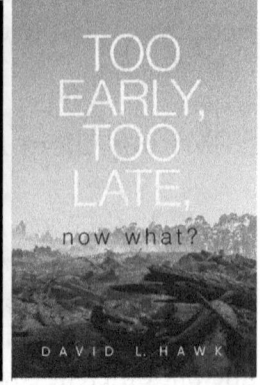
3.

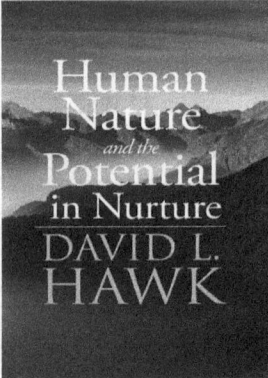
4.

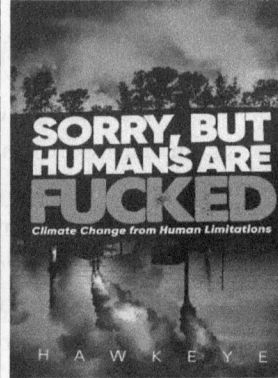
5.

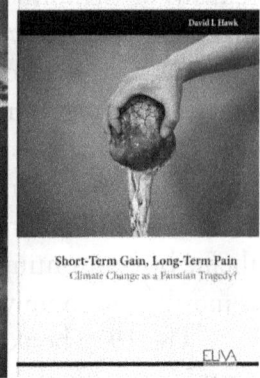
6.

The study finally came to concentrate on two nations, the USA and Sweden, as they were most different from the rest. The twenty companies were reduced to the ten generating the most pollution in the two nations from their production facilities. The people attempting to regulate in the two nations and ten companies were very helpful and came to be the major proponents of concern for climate change if human change was not created.

Wharton's Dean was upset with the three volume conclusions from the research that linked business with pollution. He was even more outspoken against: "…this climate change hoax thing." His opposition was overridden by the president of Penn who became concerned about climate change. The CEOs of Exxon and Texaco began to lecture on business changes to avoid climate change, but then were replaced by their boards who saw such as bad for business.

The situation only grew worse after the research was published and discussed. The republishing forty years later remarked on what had happened since 1979 and why it appeared to be "too late" to avoid approaching consequences of bad business. The 1979 book seemed to have no impact, except from a question from a few college professors that work in the pollution control arena: "Now that it's too late what shall we do?" In 2008 I had responded as best as I could in a university wide lecture at a school where its president had just fired me pointing out that the too late phase in problem management can be a good time to innovate with "ideas that care" as leadership with no place to go goes into hiding. The 1979 thesis was thus republished with some clarity as: *Sorry, Humans are Fucked* in late 2022 by the author "Hawkeye." The pseudonym was not at my request, nor was the qualifier "sorry."

The essence of the 1979 thesis was that in the world of actors (primarily humans) and stage sets (the context that allows human life) was about to enter a situation of reversal. Humans were traditionally cast by life as the actors that mattered with life's context organized to support their unfolding performances. Emery and Trist projected a very different situation in the human future where the "context" would become the actor of importance due to the characteristics of an industrial play that humans and written and were performing. As such the environment of human life would pass from passive to disturbed reactive then had the potential to become turbulent. As such the consequences of prior human performance would become as irreversible as the entropy process was known to be at a cosmic scale.

Therein I had described an emerging destabilized context for life where climate change consequences, as initiated by men, were becoming more important than men's capabilities to manage. Business as usual would thus become no business. that was too late to be resolved. Such grimness arose in a 1979 book on how best to regulate environmental deterioration from man's activities to enhance his life, or so he thought. The original 1979 version was printed by the Wharton School, University of Pennsylvania.

The 1979 book searched for a model of regulation that could best manage environmental deterioration problems prior to their becoming unmanageable. We were pretty pleased, even optimistic, about our proposal to move beyond the role of US trained lawyers in search of legal order via reductionistic analysis followed by arguments over what is unknown. We argued for the pursuance of a negotiated order via a non-strategic model of business that left corporate hierarchies and moved to networked organizations via computerization of communication. Companies and governments seemed to be in a collaborative mood in 1977 to 1979, as well as concerned with climate change consequences. Widespread cooperation and even collaboration was available from all involved. The results were surprising, revealing, and terrifying. Environmental deterioration via environmental desecration would destabilize the context essential for business, then for life. Contemporary regulation would be insufficient to the needs, perhaps even making things worse.

The 2022 book on humans being fucked resulted from discussions with an academic publisher that had wanted to republish the 1979 book on its 40th anniversary. They saw climate change having progressed out of being seen as a scientific hoax. The president of that university in 1979 had praised the initial report. In gratefulness I wrote a new introduction and sent it and the manuscript in for the reprinting. The book title was to be "To Early, Too Late, Now what?" One of their editors called me to say such was a very ambiguous title, that he didn't understand. He asked to know what I meant. Thus I thus sent him a new cover that I felt would offer he and others like him some direct clarity: "Humans are Fucked." He promised to never speak with me again. but described to other editors how he had defended the publishing industry against people like Hawk. One contacted me and said we would like to publish your book but would like to use the more ambiguous title. The "clear" one is a bit too clear. Too Early, Too Late, Now what? appeared in 2019. In 2021 I was contacted by a woman from another publisher saying, "It's time to go for clarity thus we would like to publish your work as "Humans are Fucked." I agreed and sent her the manuscript as rejected by the academic publisher in 2018. Without further discussion the book appeared in 2022 but with minor changes never discussed with me. The word "sorry" was to begin the title with the author given a code name of "Hawkeye" to hide any embarrassment that might occur. A third publisher then emerged and offered to republishing it with a touch of optimism. I allowed that experiment as did the first two publishers, to see if humans were okay and thus would be okay as long as they dipped into their "humanity" and fixed things. The third title became *Human Nature and the Potential in Nurture,* which did not seem to attract much attention, or attraction.

VIII

HOPELESS HUMANS,
HAPLESS HUMOR

The following outline comes from a Medium posting of about a year ago, done to collect reviewers in a common room to set a context for discussion. I repeat it here to give us a context from which to go deeper.

The movie _Bright Green Lies_, investigates the change in focus of the mainstream environmental movement, from its original concern with protecting nature, to its current obsession with powering an unsustainable way of life. The film exposes the lies and fantastical thinking behind the notion that solar, wind, hydro, biomass, or green consumerism will save us from climate change."

The increase in mining activities alone would destroy the planet. It seems to me that someone, somewhere, must be aware of this. Somehow a little of this information leaked into the psyche of the people pushing for "green" solutions. But maybe not. Maybe the folks who are trying to get everyone on board with this scheme are well meaning but deluded puppets.

I don't have a top-level security clearance or access to classified information or any "deep throat" type of informants at my beck and call, but I have this information. It seems unlikely that people in congress or people running for president would not have the same access that I do.

So what the fuck? Why aren't we being told the truth? (Do I even have to ask that?) We are not being told the truth because the truth is hellish scary, and we don't like scary. The truth would wreak havoc should it get out.

The truth about our predicament is locked up tight and not only by the folks who stand to lose a great deal if it gets out but also by your friends and neighbors and wives and husbands and boyfriends and girlfriends and everyone else you know who cannot deal with the horrible reality of the position we find ourselves in.

The crux of this issue is that no one, not you, not me, not anyone wants this party to end. We just don't. You can say that we mean well but that won't go very far when the world is burning.

In the end you are either going to believe we are in big, fat trouble or not and if not, well, you were warned.[40]

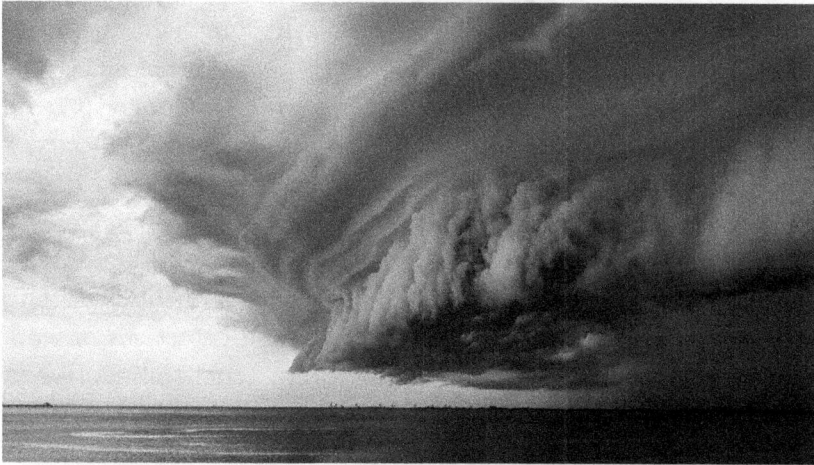

Our Real Reality

A fundamental concern that will emerge with some clarity is how will humans behave via climate change consequences, thus conditions, emerged in the everyday lives of humans? Will they seek and

---

[40] Michael Campi, "How Much, How Long, How Bad," Medium.com, Oct 30, 2022.

find alternatives to traditions and innovatively join in collaborative problem solving? Or will they dig deeper for more efficient means to kill or be killed? Closely aligned with the creating and making use of human strategy as deceit is the thinking of Adam Smith, and his sense of capitalism. Smith's fragments are bound together via the principles of Darwinian evolution, as he took them from Aristotelian logic. Smith proposed an economic attitude that could at least make it to the medium term via logical selfishness. Darwin elaborates on a means to allow this to evolve via conflict that is "logical." Aristotle, as he came to be used in computer science programming sees the logical as eternal. All three seem wrong in light of humans preparing to vacate the plant although via an evolution of means. Beginning in Constitutions, then moving to Bibles it ends in AR-15s and/ or nuclear devices. Each was seen as man's best means to preserve empires of dirt.

The idea of "hapless humans" helps us understand the emergence of "helpless humans." Hapless gains relevance in the 4th dimension as time unravels planetary life and species existence. Hapless humans lack fortune, fame, and luck. They can no longer pretend honor via an artificial status atop an ill formed Darwinian hierarchy. They act to bring calamity to themselves and their context. The above is self-generated.

Humans seem to now concentrate on maximal eating of minimal quality thus brining about 3D expansion of themselves. This occurs as they sit in front of 2D computerized depictions of work and play at home in their quest for access to better realities. When work and entertainment irritate humans go out for a car drive along lines of 1D meaning towards a 0D point of it all, thus mostly discover the pointlessness of it all. This is known as haplessness. Around the above is a collapsing context, endangered by the above human choices and actions resulting from such. Yes, humans can pull into a Starbucks to watch the news of an approaching war or generate some self-generated hatred towards those at the next table. The result is to see humans sit as "hapless" creatures.

What does hapless have to do with current progression and potential end state of the above. There are many ways to describe life's end state. For simplicity I now reference the human state as one of being fucked. Such offers the greatest clarity for the most humans. Having been working in the subject area since the nineteen seventies, while teaching at the Stockholm School of Economics, I came to see that proverbial half-filled glass of business as clearly empty. No success can be noted in humans reversing to an C cubed state, a situation of Climate Change Consequences.

August 9, 2021, Barbie Nadeau commented in the Daily Beast, "UN Climate Experts to the World: We're Already Fucked." As a code red for humanity she passed on the conclusion of a 3,949-page IPCC (UN Intergovernmental Panel on Climate Change) report. "Major new report says it is too late to stop manmade climate change – but if we act right now (fall, 2021) we could limit some of the devastation."

Adam Smith strongly believed development should be based on economics and was best supported in an environment of open competition operating in accordance with greed is good. Smith's 3 natural laws of the economics of the universe: Law of self-interest – people work for their own good. Law of competition – competition forces people to make a better product for lower price. Law of supply and demand – enough goods would be produced at the lowest price to meet the demand in a market economy." This specifically ignores, and/or opposes the universal 2nd Law of Thermodynamics. What were Adam Smith's two most important ideas? Smith's two most prominent ideas– *"invisible hand" and division of labor*–are now foundational economic theories. Both continue in the 21st century as basic to modern economic theory. In America the invisible hands belong to lobbyists divided into distinctive project domains while becoming the basis for laws as corporate employers direct.

Rule: Assume there is no misinterpretation of what is communicated, especially if it is intended as a lie. Reality can even be lower than pessimism. In 2007 I took a team of New Jersey Government and business leaders to meet in Berlin with representatives from the West and the former East Germany. There was a concluding discussion when we returned from field trips around the former East Germany. Berlin's mayor, that ran the meeting, had brought a professor of environmental law into the meeting. He gave a very gracious, and somewhat optimistic speech on what Germany had been and will do. When done the Mayor turned to me and asked if I wished to respond, as climate change consequences were known by him to be a major interest. The leader if the NJ group intervened with:

> "Please, you must understand David is a pessimistic about humans. Don't pay too much attention to any response to the wonderful presentation from this professor on environmental concerns. Hawk always sees 'glasses' as half empty, especially if they are clearly half full."

To which I responded: "Yes, but the human glass is now empty and covered in urine stains." The room then emptied.[41]

1. Beginnings, Developments, Entropic Endings

This reprints some parts of a 1977 book written to summarize a two-year project. It was in partial fulfillment of a troubled dissertation for a university degree. That book took two committees two years to review, and finally required a presidential override to pass. The subject was controversial and written in a non-dissertation manner so those who helped me in government and companies would understand.

The truth in this is funny, but reviewers did not see the humor. The Dean of the school in question found only such a symptom of my problems, with the books subject, climate change consequences, being a hoax. "How could someone invest so much in what didn't matter and wasn't?" The Head of US EPA at the time was even more upset with the contents and its challenge to his egotism.

The contents of the book outlined unhappy results from a 1975-77 study of how humans attempt to regulate their problems. Based on cooperation of six nations dealing with pollution gener-

---

[41] Based on my remark, I was later invited by the professor and mayor to give the keynote lecture to the annual Leibnitz conference that was to meet in Berlin.

ating factories and refineries of twenty companies in their national boundaries, that also provided unrestricted access, the results were pretty pessimistic. American trained lawyers came out with less esteem than the governments and companies relying on their ideas about truth. The research was into the relative effectiveness of governing environmental pollution resulting from business attempting to meet human needs and psycho wants. Hierarchies in companies and those regulating them were found to be a limitation on creative responses as well as change.

The research also documented the eternal dilemma of the US brand of politicians that got to appoint the directors of government agencies. Such choices seemed to always show an effort to please those granting political power, not achievements in the interests of the wider society. This process has long been apparent in societies. The US Senator and staff who wrote the US Water Quality Act was very helpful to the research in describing how crafty lawyers becoming politicians could avoid criticisms via writing 10,000-page laws filled with 100-word sentences about requirements as well as their opposites near the end. This was said to come from a law school education where students are to see there to be laws and ethics, where you will be more successful in confining the arguments to the first and avoid the second.

The Swedish approach showed the greatest difference of the other five nations. It was based on all environmental laws taking up 25 pages. The director of their regulation efforts responded to the conclusions of the study: "We Swedes seem a bit strange, compared to the US. We strongly feel the precondition to obeying a law is to understand it." More important to the results was that all the facilities of companies in the study had cleaner results than they did in the US, and almost no litigation over innovative ideas for achieving such.

What we call business activities, presumably based on economic theories, have come to change the contexts of life. The 1979 book was very concerned with this and discussed changes to ideas of business, ideologies of economics, and valuation of our contexts. The book ended with concern for life from impending and expanding threats from climate change consequences. Significant changes in attitudes, practices and methods of governance were outlined. Industry scientists described how climate change would come to redefine the context of life. Parts of the original study will be found herein as abstracted.

While the arrangement of words found herein are first to improve my own understanding of where we are at and how we got here. It is then hoped that others will come to find these contents helpful to their understanding of what many were told is too complex for non-experts to understand, or already being taken care of by those who know. Both attitudes are wrong while the change needed is urgent. Tomorrow is almost too late. The emphasis in the study was how best to support bio-needs, while working to modify psycho-wants. Those funny billionaire types are mostly ignored as they mostly ignore the importance of context, a context they endanger, in feeding their psycho-wants at the price of the context required for life. Besides, they are mostly concentrated on implications of the movie "Don't Look Up," thus planning to get to Mars as life on earth ends so they need not engage in the planetary death march of live that remains as they move on from their mistakes. Just now they are mostly involved in creating an approach to artificial intelligence that will do a final battle with what remains of natural intelligence. intelligence.

The prior edition had a very clear title, but some clearly needed it to not be while almost appreciating the content. It may be worthwhile to introduce the history of entitling a common theme of mine from 1979 until 2023. I believe this helps outline the meaning and substance of the stories found in all these books. Please keep in mind that the following was written to me to attempt understand what is unfolding, and if it has meaning. If you find any sign of deeper than usual understanding about life I will greatly appreciate you. Yes, just as you know I will know. If you find the contents offensive to who and what you are, such as that offensive tree that attempts to grow in your backyard without your permission I will also understand that.

I have three daughters that are on my mind as I write. I hope they excuse my limits as I attempt to understand our collective future. I understand that my former wives do not excuse my idiot behavior as I attempted to deal with short-term gains while understanding there are long-term pains, in the Faustian sense of how we make a mess of life.

Business, who and what directs it, is important to 21st Century humans as most costs be levied against the planet are incurred from business transactions. The taking of risks via innovation is not the problem, as humans have always been noted for such. Much success is derived from such. The issue in this book is what from the seventh century on there was an exaggeration in how the innovators and their managers need not pay the price for their mistakes in doing so. The costs for error were sent to lower parts of the societal hierarchy or laid as waste in a seemingly unresponsive nature.

I ran an architectural design studio at Iowa State University with the focus being on the effect of the 2nd Law of Thermodynamics on products of building creation and maintenance. The following diagram of such was done by some students. They saw this as the selfish concern of business as usual in the design firm, where the higher you were in the hierarchy of control the more you followed this problem-solving flow. Their alternative was seen in leadership choices from 1850 in setting the tone for industrialization of providing for human food and shelter.

This diagram was from a 1981 studio at Iowa State University, where students were beginning to be realistic about the mental conditions of their elders in pursuance of business as usual. Students even changed the design studio, replacing sealed windows with operatable ones, to make it more accommodating to life while lessoning the building's contribution to entropy.

The president of Iowa State University was upset with students relating to this diagram as a way to get architectural designs approved, then constructed. Students argued that something more ethical and longer-term was needed. The students were unhappy with the measures of success used in the building they occupied and were to learn from. They said the new design center was a further step down the road to the artificial as non-natural, even anti-natural. As such students felt they must act to critic if not improve the ISU building. The president felt Professor Hawk was at the center of the students changing the building. Hawk was more at the perimeter commenting that the new Design Center was a continuation of the theme from 1850 for an ever-expanding *business as usual* process of the industrial against the natural, heavily dependent on use of ever more energy in buildings that left nature out. Regardless, the President fired Hawk for using diagrams like the one below to outline principles of business as usual.

Normal Problem-Solving Flows

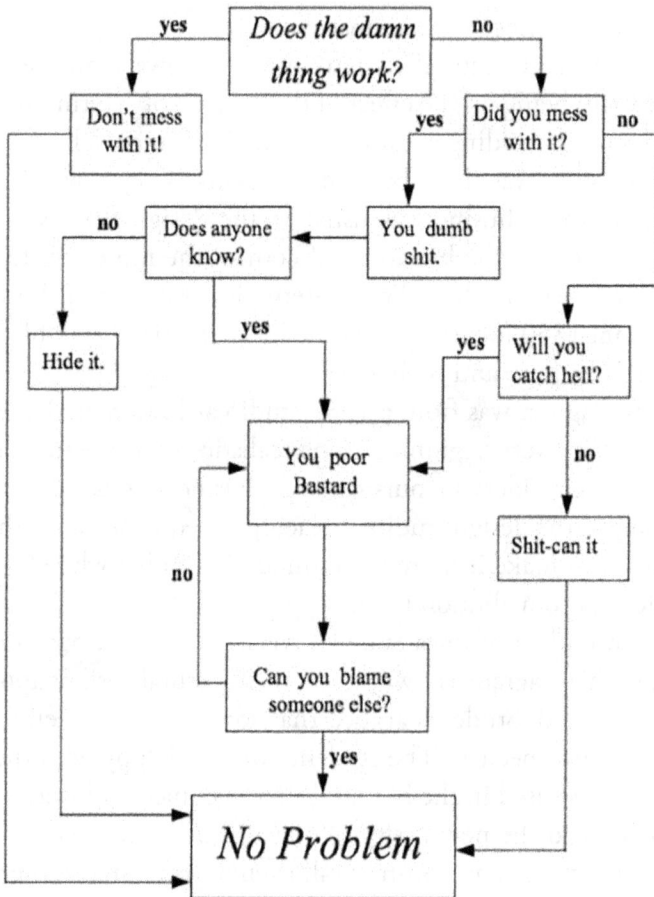

Source: Unknown

I agreed with his being upset with my arguments against business as usual becoming no business via climate change consequences. I had encouraged students to seek ways to soften the pending consequences of climate change from doing what had been normal since 1850. I encouraged *business as unusual,* which was not well-understood, except in some leading companies. Universities and their leaders were clueless of such change and any need for it.

2. Eunice Newton Foote, A Light Men Couldn't See

In 1979 my concern for the future became clearer. It was written in the four volume conclusions from a 2-year study as aided by twenty companies and six nations. Its point was to see how, or even if, we could regulate environmental destruction from humans being human. From the study results we could show how pollution, from industrialization of human needs and psycho wants, would expand until it modified that thin layer of planetary life support until life was not. Our conclusions came to be consistent with early knowledge of Eunice Newton Foote, who in 1856 published a science paper on how expanding CO^2 from energy used for industrialization would reduce life. She modelled the process for generating atmospheric heat from the pollution resulting from coal-fired power plants.

While she was completely ignored by men and largely ignored by society, she came to be unknown by being right. I was introduced to her work by a chief scientist of Exxon who showed me her 120-year-old work on climate change. I also saw her work in support of women's rights and suffrage movements articulated by her colleague Susan B. Anthony. She saw how masculine values in a particular model of industrialization would bring danger to life. She was quite right, sadly. Elsewhere I use her work to argue against our current models of leadership and management, especially the values derived from the first three letters of management.

We have now moved on another 44 years from the 1979 work. Little change and no progress has taken place in turning from our confrontation with a natural reality created in praise of an artificial stage set of humans. Research results from the 1975-77 study, as documented in our 1979 book, were presented to OECD membership and many others. The consequences of badly managed industrialization as described in our research have only expanded.

Do humans care? Is our leadership defective, or do we choose such leaders so we can avoid responsibility and sleep between our checking on bank balances? Whatever keeps humans from radically changing to meet ominously approaching threats is our concern herein. It appears that humans are indeed "fucked," as that very old expression of situations goes. Is this due to lack of intelligence, laziness of spirit, or meanness? To understand this question, we need to look at our situation and its assumptions for a disaster.

I used to give lectures on "The potential in its Too Late." I would argue how humans learn best from experiencing the most difficult challenges, conditions, and consequences. In my lectures I would offer examples of the cost of bad leadership, humans knowing it was bad, but still tolerating it until it seemed too late. Once it's too late the leaders, those who try to lead but have no place to go, disappear. They go into hiding, or to Mars or the Moon, to avoid the consequences of their actions. Once gone there is a small chance to accomplish much in radically different activities from those who care. In the seventies I documented this in companies whose incompetent boards would seek out men like Texas Chainsaw Al Dunlap to openly lead them into irrelevance then bankruptcy. Noteworthy was that Wall Street loved them and their forceful actions to show strength. In those studies, done at the Wharton School of Business we came to classify the employees that didn't need such leadership, but tolerated it, as being "fucked." We seem to be in a global version of the same tragedy.[42]

Concern for improving human capabilities in life seems to be growing. It is most urgent in youth via growing disassociation with future living. It can be seen in growing anger towards adults as well as in adults with anger at others in their way and self as creators of climate change conditions. With greater frequency humans consider

---

[42] "A Study of Scott Paper Company: From demonstrating how leadership gets in the way of innovative employees to the hiring of Al Dunlap to destroy it all." Wharton School Publications, Social Systems Sciences Program, 1975.

suicide plus take note of projects, products and people failing to live up to promises in ads or from CEOs. While passing through the fourth-dimension projects, products and people seem to degrade, then dissolve. Ads and commercials that brought us to them tend to be provided overtly optimistic in time. Via growth in consequences of climate change we note such more systematically. A large collection of products are combined in a systemic conclusion for life using them or occupying context near them. A growing array of species of life are disappearing. Those remaining alive encounter death threats from viruses and chemicals. Each day the life we depend on to support our life is vanishing from the planet or watching its context replaced with rising waters or storms not experienced in hundreds of years. As we listen to expanding lies from our governments and leaders our hope seems limited to lies.

In an optimistic streak Cohen suggests there is hope in the crackage developing in human systems. Crackage management of deadly processes allows us to move from seeking the causes of our consequences. We begin to develop ways to see future effects of current effects instead of suspending our vision via burying our heads in the sand seeking the historical causes of those contemporary effects. Humans can now begin to see the cracks in our systems and then better understand where the consequences of such move. Considering the qualities, or lack thereof, in what humans do can find hope in looking for and repairing problems behind the cracks. Avoiding such mostly comes from acting out our egocentric beliefs in human having ultimate control over nature, as well as other items, e.g., other humans. What are the barriers to seeing the cracks and the light coming through the cracks?

Humans seem incapable of seeing the predictable downfalls from what they market as products of our rational perfection. This is especially apparent in what humans do to create what is displayed as omnipresence in human industrialization, a technological pathway of what we like to call humanism. This began in religions designed to soften the enigma of life, necessarily ending in death. With time we found death-insulating religions to protect us. Often these ran counter to knowledge creating religions called science.

3. The Arrogance of Humanism

Omnipotence moved from life after death, to eroding death via life of humanists. Ehrenfeld effectively argued that there were cracks in a long trail of humanistic lore, where light of a richer truth lay behind such cracks. The following is a partial explanation presented in his 1973 work.

During the years of the rise of humanism there were powerful voices, indeed humanist voices, which, if heeded, might have diminished the arrogant tendency, inherited from the old religions, to believe in our ability to manipulate the earth in many ways and to avoid paying any ultimate penalties for this manipulation. As Clarence Glacken has noted, and Francis Bacon, Kant, Hume, and Goethe all warned – in different ways and to different degrees – about the weaknesses and dangers inherent in the doctrine of final causes, and about the problems that it would create. But these voices were not heeded.

> In fact, Bacon's celebrated phrase "Nature is only to be commanded by obeying her." Even if the context of Bacon's comment was from a brand of limited arrogance, he has been ignored in more ways by more people than any other source of intelligent ideas of our times. Today one can still find a few humanists, such as Lewis Mumford, trying patiently to explain that Nature is not like a machine. Indeed, Mumford cites Kant's argument that a machine contains an external organizing principle while Nature does not. But these few are outnumbered and outshouted by a multitude that prefers to cling to simple-minded analogies which confirm its faith in the ability of humans to solve any puzzle, overcome any obstacle, and fulfill any quest.[43]

---

[43] David Ehrenfeld, *The Arrogance of Humanism*, New York: Oxford University Press, 1978, p. 8-9

Serious problems, leading to fateful costs, are hidden behind the puffery and arrogance of human behavior. Cohen's idea of there being crackage can be seen in most products built from an arrogance of knowing what cannot be known. The cracks are a sign of optimism after the arrogance fades from fear. With cracks you can see locations for improvement while dampening homocentric arrogance. His deep concern for the road humans choose to travel is seen in his poetry.

Such comments seem consistent with mental disorders clearly expressed in the movie "Catch 22," and perhaps even more so in Bateson's idea of wrongful communication in schizophrenic families such as with the mother who bought two neckties for her young son, one blue, one green. In the story of such we begin to see the hopelessness of the digital, the tired twosomes in mental health.

> The next day the child is in a hurry to sport the green necktie. The mother: 'So you don't like the blue tie I gave you?' The next day the boy puts on the blue tie and draws the symmetrical response: 'So you don't like the green tie I gave you?' So, on the third day, the child tried to find a compromise solution in order to satisfy his mother's two demands: he puts on the two ties together. And his mother comments: 'You poor boy, you're out of your mind. You're going to drive me crazy.'[44]

Herein the digital challenges of climate change consequences is seen as a key motivator for humans to change in order to locate improvements essential to continuance. In the 1970's research project by Hawk, et.al, discovered how regulations designed by Americans to control environmental degradation from manufacturing contained the essence of Bateson "double binds." Economic developed must be furthered by improved productivity of that which created pollution regardless of varieties and qualities of pollution. One set of regulations against toxic waste in one American state was truly schizo-

---

[44] G Bateson, Paul Watzlawick, Jackson, Haley and Weakland, "Toward a Theory of Schizophrenia," *Behavior Science*, 1, 251-254, 1956.

phrenic in that it outlawed toxic waste by demanding their nonexistence thus making the court-based debates very clear, and clearly deranged. Judges and the companies they were judging faced double binds. The situation of avoiding climate change effects now seen fifty years later is clearly a double bind, and doorway to the schizophrenic.

Bateson was captured by the idea of "double binds," especially those self-defined to allow unanswerable contradictions in life. He added science to "damned if you do, damned if you don't." He demonstrated how human endeavors can include activities in religions, politics, sciences, housing, foods, transporting and relationships with others, and with their environments. I advocated change while religious beliefs, being from and of culture, illustrated changelessness.[45] While some marvel at that which is crack free, technologically, I smile and tell them to just wait, nature will have her way. For improvement of life I would look for signs of crackage, especially those hard to see. I became known for seeing cracks that others said were not there but did get fired quite often by leadership and management seen to emphasize crackage repair. They were uncomfortable in my describing the differences between leadership and leadershit, then pointing out their emphasis in masculinity measures as thought to lie with penis size; imaginary or real. Perhaps they were/are most upset with my belief that our poorly performing industrial needs to experiment with leadership via feminine values. Perhaps this would be called *Femagement*.

[45] David Hawk, Satu Teerikangas, Annaleena Parhankangas, Taina Ikonen, "Changelessness, and Other Impediments to Systems Performance & Management," Proceedings of: *World Multi-conference on Systems, Cybernetics and Informatics*, Orlando, Florida. 2001.

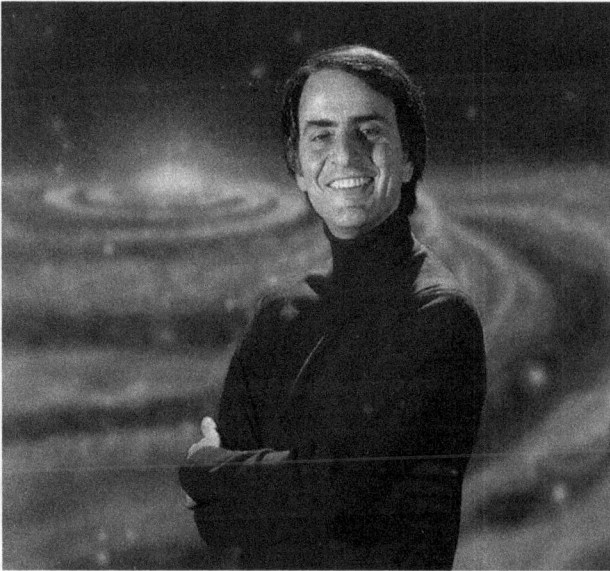

1980: Carl Sagan, Concern with Human Bullshit

"One of the saddest lessons of history is this: If we've been bamboozled long enough, we tend to reject any evidence of the bamboozle. We're no longer interested in finding out the truth. The bamboozle has captured us. It's simply too painful to acknowledge, even to ourselves, that we've been taken. Once you give a charlatan power over you, you almost never get it back."[46]

This was well stated in a 2005 Princeton University Press publication. It looked like a tiny black book as composed by a Harry G. Frankfurt, Professor Emeritus of Philosophy, Princeton University. Titled *On Bullshit*, it became a best-seller in the Princeton University Bookstores. A decade later is became a symbol of how a Donald Trump became an acceptable leader to America, standing on bullshit.

---

[46] Carl Sagan, from a tape of a joint presentation he and I made in a Conference in Canada in 1980 by the World Futures Organization. We talked of the Cosmos, Climate Change Research, and Entropy as fundamental.

One of the most salient features of our culture is that there is so much bullshit. Everyone knows this. Each of us contributes his share. ....Bullshit is unavoidable whenever circumstances require someone to talk without knowing what he is talking about. Thus the production of bullshit is stimulated whenever a person's obligations or opportunities to speak about some topic exceed his knowledge of the facts that are relevant to that topic. ...Rather than seeking primarily to arrive at accurate representations of a common world, the individual turns towards trying to provide honest representations of himself. Convinced that reality has no inherent nature, which he might hope to identify as the truth about things, he devotes himself to being true to his own nature. It is as though he decides that since it makes no sense to try to be true to the facts, he must therefore try instead to be true to himself.[47]

In 2015, a candidate for US Presidency, Donald Trump, would talk with some affection about bags of lies. With time some would come to call his bags bullshit. In this regard when I was teaching business leadership courses I would recommend a 2005 book by a Professor of Philosophy at Princeton University. Titled *On Bullshit* it was very helpful as a text to prepare for the American future. It was a good entry into discussions of the weaknesses of what in 2006 was being taught in leading business programs relative to strategic thinking and marketing as necessarily dishonest business endeavors in the short-term. It was then hoped that the longer-term cost could be discounted.

Even the 1832 articulator of strategic thinking in the conduct of warfare, Carl von Clausewitz, explained why strategy must be deceit to be effective in the 19th Century. The consequences of such are sad. Leadership should be restricted to the time of an operational task as needed by a group, and that such a person is very good at. When

---

[47] Harry G. Frankfurt, *On Bullshit*, Princeton, NJ: Princeton University Press, 2005, pp. 1, 63-64.

completed leadership moves on to another who is especially killed at the next necessary task. Permanent leadership is a simple-minded and usually shameful path into a human immortality project while knowing death awaits. In other work I point out how this is consistent with the very powerful underlying intellectual argument for climate change. With entropy as the infinite process behind climate change the extensive advertising of its non-existence my best be seen as "negative entropy." Such avoided the beauty and pain of reality by adds and speeches that promise no cost, no pain and access to immortality via the product or process.

Returning to the Cohen wisdom of song I noted how my observation of cracks in human systems was central to accessing the differences that ended up making the difference. For each crack, as I would comment on it, came to have a price associated with it. Even though I might be richly rewarded later I would need to pay an admission price to the discourse; usually seen in my being openly fired to encourage others to be obedient. Much of my work, mostly called advisement or building, came to be advocating for more *business as unusual*. Cracks were initially noted in assumptions that then underlay *business as usual*.

In what follows I mention some of my life's low points, those which appeared as shit in my life-long fight against such. As you review these points I trust you will see where I'm not especially different from you, and most other humans. My major problem proved to be me. I was a bit too open in my language choices in commenting on and suggestion needed change. I was said to be scary, but I doubt I was. I also was not very strong, just didn't know what to do and assumed what was most wrong was me.

Scary people do not give half their income to others, such as helping students pay their tuition costs or donating more than half my income to charities that attempt to help. I found that it was hard to maintain grades in college when I was working from 8PM to 4 AM loading trucks for UPS, then attempting to stay awake in classes. From being around my mother I found that women and children needed to find ways to compensate for men that were someplace else. After scanning my trek through life I have thought more about how bad others have it, and think it was best to just tolerating what is not understandable. Just now humanity is in a similar situation in beginning to experience climate change consequences in daily negotiation with existence. If our perceptions are confused or clouded it is easy to look at articles of the 95% of scientists that study climate change.

Next time you want to be alone in your thoughts and go out driving, e.g., today, think about the items you are thinking about, and how those change. For example, when I was seven, and working on the farm, I was expected to drive tractors, trucks, and cars. Sometimes it was on a 15-mile trek between two farms we were farming. As I drove at age seven, I would wave to other drivers in a sense of friendliness, but also in pride that he and I were similar in our high status. We were "drivers." Ten years later, when we would meet while driving, we had moved up to raising a first finger and smile to each other, all in appreciation of our joint positions and occupations in life.

In another ten years we had graduated, or the world had changed, to expect our giving each other our middle fingers to symbolize that each of us owned the road and didn't appreciate their using it. Now, after another twenty years many in Iowa now exercise their Trump-like salute to gain respect or illustrate our deep concern for our "Second Amendment Rights and First Amendment Freedoms." We just keep on getting better, right? What does this mean for 2024?

Soon we may realize that human activities, such as driving around using up gas while looking for truth and privacy, is a part of how humans come to damage our planet. The conditions we generate while driving tend to upset the context on which life depends. Clearly the fossil fuels used to drive is one of the major contributors to climate change. How can we has humans change all this? Next time we go out for a drive and have the radio on listening to a book on our radio, say a book about humans ending life on their planet, we can begin to think of our options for making the planet livable for the children. How does that sound? The more we drive and think the better we can feel, until we can't feel. This book is about such, and such humans, including me, and the way I somehow live here on my farm in Iowa. Sorry, this is getting pretty heavy. Maybe I need to go for a drive, to relax and feel like I'm in charge of it all.

Yes, I have experiences with "Cracks in Human Systems," systems I helped create and maintain as well as some of the crackage. The alternative is normal problem solving, as seen in students' thinking based on what is taught within MBA courses, and reference books.

4. Faustian Bargaining, With Our Inner-Selves

In a 2022 book, *Short-Term Gain, Long-Term Pain: Climate Change as a Faustian Tragedy*, I addressed the question of – "What now?" – that ended a 2019 book, *Too Early, Too Late, What now?*

The 2022 book confronted European man's hundreds of years battling between his doing what was right, for the longer-term and the context, or simply being more immediate and jumping into short-term acquisitions of silly wealth, wrong knowledge, and beautiful sex mates. The short-term does have costs but they seem trivial on a day-to-day basis, especially when compared to the beauty of potential sex mates. Thus, most men suspended any concern for the long-term until it's too late. In their beginnings they argued: "We are all dead in the long-term so why bother?" The best way I knew of discussing the resulting problems, usually very serious to life, and its context was via a 15th Century concept of Faustian Bargaining to define the manly attitude.

One of the greatest literary heroes, Johann Wolfgang von Goethe, was born in Frankfurt am Main, Germany on August 28, 1749. Much of his writing was simply a masterpiece for humans and me to better understand human thinking than behavior. I was fond of his work "The Eternal Feminine," and named a Chinese Foundation of mine in its honor. Most agree his foremost work was in his development of the Faustian tragedy as plays, Parts I and II.

I was fascinated with this at several levels. The most superficial was with one of my Swedish relatives was Cori Faust, born in Smoland, Sweden October 1819. She was a cousin of Gustaf Oscar Schillerstrom born in Kalmar, Sweden Feb 02, 1817. Gustaf moved to America in his youth and died in my country, Jefferson County,

Iowa April 23, 1911. He lived near a church in the village of New Sweden and wrote notes about the issues of and person Faust. As such I was interested in this Faustian issue early in my life. He would tell the story of Faust for his own religious reasons. I came to find reasons to explain its use and human reliance on such without the need for religion. For most it was the dilemma of short-term gain then long-term pain, or verse visa…ha..ha.

Faust, Faustus, or Doctor Faustus was the central figure on one of the most durable legends we can find in the folklore and/or literature of the west. There are counterparts in the East but not as widespread nor enduring. The storyline focuses on a man who is an astrologer who sells his soul to the devil. In return he receives knowledge and power or has access to what represents those. The story is said to begin in the 16th Century via Dr. Johann Georg Faust (1466 until 1540). He was an itinerant alchemist, astrologer, and magician in Germany.

Faust was first translated into a dramatization by Christopher Marlowe in 1604 via the play The Tragical History of Doctor Faustus. Outside of Shakespeare this play raised more controversy than any other in Elizabethan history of plays. The play is to show the person choosing material gains (via the devils acting to suit his desires) well over those from the spirit. It's a tough version of Faust where during much of his life he does nothing worthwhile as serving as a university scholar he tells those around him that he is damned for what he had gained but is unsure if it was worthwhile. When he dies the devil's messenger comes to collect the soul by dismembering the body.

The next version of Faust, probably the most memorable one, came from Goethe. Faust was an obsession of Goethe for almost sixty years. The story comes in two parts. In the first part Faust makes a deal with the devil to attain the zenith of happiness, prior to collecting the soul. As with most humans since, Faust believes the moment of death will never come. Part I lays out a story of a not very great experience ending in a lustful and destructive relationship with a beautiful and innocent girl named Gretchen. As part of the story the devil destroys Gretchen and her family by deceptions, desires, and bad actions. Part I ends with a reversal where Gretchen is saved, and

Faust goes off into shame. In Part II Faust was reconstituted by the earth's spirits and meets politicians, classical gods and even Helen of Troy (the image of the world's most beautiful women). As Faust dies the devil reaches for the soul but the Lord intervenes and carries him to heaven as he found Faust very resourceful and always striving.

Thomas Mann then wrote *Doktor Faustus* in the 1950's, for which he received a Nobel Prize, but I prefer the version of 1945 as written at the end of WWII. That was where its author looked at the devastation around him from the war and posed that the devil and his assistants all moved underground in complete fear of humans. Yes, humans were out to sell their soul but at any price. The getting rid of the soul was more important than the price.

IX

1975-77: DEEPER INTO THAT SWEDISH RESEARCH PROJECT

A two-year Stockholm research project was conducted into the above concerns relative to if and how such could be regulated by government. The project came to focus on two ways to regulate it. As such it went well beyond the tradition of doing studies of the effectiveness of pieces of regulation to examine the chances for success of analytic (short term) partial responses to systemic (longer-term consequential) difficulties. The results from the two years of work were clarifying yet troubling. This document attempts to present and explain these results.

The research was set up to examine the role of relationships in leading to long-term consequences of human acts. The relationships were between humans, between humans and nature, then between humans and their images of themselves. All the relations were analyzed with a clearly rational emphasis on cause-effect understanding of parts. This non-systemic approach was taken to help understand the mentality behind the actions, not the systemic consequences of those actions. That was examined later. The non-systemic was found to be based in a desire for stability via the values of changelessness. An alternative value set emerged from participants at the edge of

142

operations; those who lived in a world of change. As a sign of there being a better way towards problem resolution the results of the study point to the clarity of views coming from the edges; those who embraced change and practiced fluid management of connections, not parts. Those bound by analysis could only see parts, not connections. Those thinking systemically came to mostly see connections while overlooking behavior of parts. As such, the project focus became critical of standard economic thinking, acting, and managing. It was useful to show how humans arrive at valuations, especially what they value more than life.

Humans seem to be developing what is herein called the *human project.* In its essence, the current stage of development is seen to be based in Newtonian-directed industrialization values. These seek the mechanical rationality that can be seen in emphasizing causal results from backward analysis of effects. Herein this is seen as 1-dimensional greed managed by regulating within the limits of 2-dimensional thoughts on paper. Ostensibly, the purpose of the human project is to supply human needs with reduced human work all while encouraging humans to seek fulfillment in life through inventing and seeking material wants.

Meanwhile, humans tend to not notice, or not care, about the peripheral costs in the ever-expanding human project's environmental deterioration from one–dimensional thinking as seen in three-dimensional danger to life. This, added to the irreversible nature of natural entropic deterioration, pose serious problems for systems of living order. Early responses to this, by those humans who notice something amiss, is, once again, 1-dimensional ideas set out on 2-dimensional paper to manage the complexities of 3-dimensional deterioration. Those who seem to most understand the situation see all this as *a band aid awaiting surgery.*

1. Overview of the Human Situation

The ways in which we conceive of and relate to our environments are being challenged and changed. They clearly need to be. Some social systems are experimenting with replacement guides to 19th and 20th century ideals and mythologies which have driven social industrialization. Industrial products have significantly improved the human condition, but also generated a waste stream of simmering natural and social problems that still await resolution. Continuing expansion of the same industrial model is now failing to meet even the underlying economic assumptions and expectations. If we continue unchecked, we will encounter climate change consequences as noted in the 1975-77 research project based at the Stockholm School of Economics, which several of those involved in this work were also involved.

Those caught up in the consequences of traditional industrial process are in deep trouble. This is creating a small and growing movement to change priorities, such as shifting from managing the effects of industrialization to managing the values that define and drive it. In this way it, or a replacement version of it, might come to be redefined, redesigned, and revalued. This becomes especially urgent as the less-developed parts of the world now rush to place their stakes on the table of economic development via industrialization. China is now the prime example. Their joining into the industrial development game raises the level of urgency for improving our myths and models of global economic development.

Not only should the business-as-usual model not be expanded to other nations, but its previous level of activity also cannot be sustained in those relying upon it, and its products are no longer clearly linked to human well-being. Even the underlying economic assumptions that it will provide for increasing employment are faltering. Its central flaw appears to be that its success is contingent upon continuous expansion. It contains no homeostatic mechanism at its core that accommodates stabilization. This is why political discussions of the need to "shift" to a more "sustainable model" of development are not especially innovative for the present, nor attractive for the future. Their underlying assumptions must hinge on a reality of sustainability of continued growth, not sustainability of the human environment.

This can be seen in the extreme level of competition between international firms over being given access to China's economic development agenda. They must grow to survive globally. Only those companies that are now redefining their development models, and the design of the supporting infrastructures, are not worried about Chinese markets. Some of these were included in the study. Very interesting and beneficial alternatives to business-as-usual do exist but are not widely known nor discussed.

New metaphors and models of how products should be designed and produced for human uses are needed. These tap into the need for individualized redevelopment programs, instead of continuation of external societal development. This is the difference between single-copy and mass forms of production and consumption. The advantages of new design and production process for the human condition can now be seen in the R&D recesses of several companies. Some of these are described in the report. They are sufficiently exciting and advanced to call for shifting from traditional concerns with what to do, towards why it isn't being done.[48] Some of the R&D output has even moved discussion why more isn't being done to how to better manage the creative minds that will be bringing these new visions of product forming and use into society? The subject of this report is thus product innovation and its management.

The product concept includes design and production with less emphasis on arguments over which is most important to environmental values. Some technical and product specifics are presented, but only to give the management subject matter a clear sense of its overriding objective - improved relations between humans and their environments. This requires a reconceptualization of the term environment, and the various environments in which humans live and work.

---

[48] This theme came up repeatedly in the research during interviews of the most innovatively experienced people working on environmental concerns. In fact, the people who used this phrase were almost always in organizations perceived as the most advanced in their environmental accomplishments. Innovatively experienced means that they have invested many years in swimming against the rush of the environmental mainstream in their countries and organizations, and just now are being given a freer reign in their work and experimentations.

There are three major types of environments in which humans simultaneously live. The first is the *built* environment. Pronounced changes are taking place in how we conceptualize, produce, and relate to it. Evidence of failures in this most artificial of arenas suggests that improvements in relations to the more natural environment may be even more difficult to come by. We have designed and built artificial environments to specifically shelter and nurture human activities yet somehow, they often ended up being transformed into manifestations of human distrust and hatred. If we have such difficulties relating to the environments over which we have high control, then what does this imply for success in relations to environments over which we have less control? A response that forms the core of the management system recommended in this report is that control may be the wrong issue.

The second environmental type is more elusive and fundamental. It is the bio-physical context from which we come, on which we rely for life, and to which we return upon death. We know it as the *natural* environment. For three hundred years the American conception of nature has been shifting. To the pilgrim's nature was a location that offered dangers, yet great promise. To the puritan's nature was the wilderness of lust, evil and ungodliness.[49] Later arrivals the new world perceived the natural environment as a resource reservoir, although they also ended up carrying some of their puritan ancestor's baggage. More recent descendants have turned nature it into a dis-

---

[49] Others have defined a puritan as one who goes through life with a funny, nagging suspicion that someone, somewhere is having a good time, and they don't like. Several European authors have pointed to our Puritan beginnings as a reason for what they see as a flaw in the American character. They illustrate this by pointing out how we fear seeing nakedness on TV, in outdoor advertisements or on beaches, yet have exceptional tolerance for physical violence.

posal dump and then a phenomenon of fear,[50] Only recently is it seen as a possible base for renewal of the human condition.[51]

The third environment may be the most important, and most challenging. This is the sphere of influence we know as the *social* environment. It too is being changed as part of an ongoing societal flux in how we perceive each other and how we live and work with, or against, each other. Most of the dilemmas of the human condition can be found in this arena. They may begin within the individual psyche, but they get manifested in the social conditions. Our activities in the social environment illustrate the potentials and dilemmas of the human condition. As we move towards greater connectedness to others, by making cities and other social institutions, we long for more insulated and isolated from others in our houses and hearts. The way in which we resolve these dilemmas with economic and political acts in our social environment will be critical to how we

---

[50] One means to see this is in the writings of Y-fu Chan, a professor of geography, such as *Topophilia* and *Landscapes of Fear*, Pantheon Books: New York, 1979. He describes how the landscapes of fear change as we and societies age. "We watch as human beings continually draw and redraw their 'circles of safety,' never feeling entirely at peace with them."(cover sheet)

[51] An access point into this idea is seen in the writings of the late biologist Rene Dubos, especially in his 1981 *Celebrations of Life*, and 1980 *The Wooing of Earth*, Charles Scribner's Sons: New York. He shows how humans have both despoiled and embellished nature. "With our knowledge and a sense of responsibility for the welfare of humankind and the Earth, we can create new environments that are ecologically sound, aesthetically satisfying, economically rewarding, and favorable to the continued growth of civilization. But the wooing of the Earth will have a lasting successful outcome only if we create conditions in which both humankind and the Earth retain the essence of their wildness."(p.159.) In 1986 an argument was presented that developing a new perspective towards natural resource use, one that looked at such resources as highly valuable and to be used as efficiently as possible, could be the best possible basis for a new approach to industrial design and production by US companies. It was argued that this would be a viable base for international competitiveness of products. At that time the logic was found distasteful in the economics community. See my chapter "Powering the American Eagle: The US Energy Myth and Its Probable Consequences," in *U.S. - Mexican Economic Relations*, Ed. Khosrow Fatemi, 1988.

improve our relations to the natural environment. We must find improved ways to manage our relations to each other and ourselves.

Our relations within the social environment establish the pre-conditions of how we choose to relate to other environments. This is seen in how different interest groups end up perceiving and acting out attitudes towards the subject of environmental protection.

- Lawyers want their skill to be of even more use in the field's problems.
- Engineers want to know why they aren't more used to make solutions.
- Scientists want to know why they are being used for the purposes of lawyers, environmentalists, and politicians.
- Businesspeople want to know what they can start.
- Environmentalists want to know what they can stop.
- Politicians want to know where the "movement" is going, so they can be out in front of it.
- The public wants to know what is wrong with all of the above as they walk out to the curb to recycle their bottles and papers.

This points to the underlying problem in the social environment and indicates from where the solution to natural environmental problems will need to begin. Each of the above interests has become increasingly cynical about the activities of the others, and about the initial subject of interest - the natural environment. Just now it is unclear if the measures being taken, primarily driven by lawyer politicians, are for improvement or further dismemberment of the connections between humans and their environments. We dislike the cities that we have built, yet we tend to further destroy natural environments by building new cities in our flight from what we have previously built.

Public interest (those who see the trash on the commons) and private economic interests (those who see an economic advantage in putting it there) have begun to lower some of their animosity towards each other. They mutually agree that the commons is a mess and that current governmental policies are both inefficient and ineffective in managing it. This has encouraged some tentative policy experiments with how to shift private economic interests towards public improvement. Commodity trading venues, marketing rights ventures and a myriad of self-centered economic incentives are being added to increasing public education and community-based recycling programs. This is placed on top of traditional policies of prohibitive laws, not in parallel to, or in place of.

The study was initiated in Winter, 1992 to attempt to make it through this minefield of environmental issues. Sponsored by the US EPA and the Integrated Pollution Prevention Initiative at NJIT the study was designed to examine the potentials in the variable of business management methods for helping to attain environmental objectives. The general objective was to generate information that could be used in the management education so the students might see how it was in the interest of their corporations and themselves to find better fits with their decisions, and the environmental consequences of the decisions.

For a variety of reasons, the emphasis turned to management practices in non-US firms. One rationale was that most schools already teach a great deal about US management practices, and simply adding to this load would not be attractive. Linked to this was the rationale that in the future the only business would be international business thus anything environmental management could do to align itself with international business was attractive. And finally, this was the domain where the PI of the study did most of his work.

The means to collect this information on foreign company operations and their management centered on interviews of key executives. The interviews came to focus on the R&D and product development/design aspects of linking future market possibilities to future corporate products. How these somewhat ambiguous functions are managed and should be managed in the future has become a major topic in business schools and practice. The core of the study report presents this information.

Additional activities were undertaken in parallel to see how specific students and managers could be encouraged to do things in a more reflective, innovative manner. The first stage of this was to initiate activities that would encourage students and managers to be more reflective about the dangers, complexities and opportunities in environmental sensitivity. This included paper in a conference journal, several lectures to specialized groups of students or managers, supplemental lectures in traditional management courses, and experiential visits to see what actual companies were attempting to do and actually doing with regard to environmental concerns. It is concluded that these activities have an ascending order of importance for making a difference. The papers remain mostly unread, the lectures are mostly forgotten, with memory of course content mostly lost except for the most graphic examples. The two most effective activities to get people to look more deeply into environmental concern and change their direction based on what they learned were:

- Undergraduate honors students doing paid research to present the state of the art of environmental developments in their chosen discipline to the other students. These were students from engineering, biomechanics, mathematics, and architecture.
- Graduate executive management students taking a trip to visit foreign companies that were pursuing the development of environmental technologies. These were students in upper-middle level management positions that were enrolled in a special bi-weekly program paid for by their companies.

Additional impacts seem to be emerging from the participants to the study. They have become more knowledgeable and interested in what each other is doing to develop environmental policies and practices. A few have made trips to visit each other based on comments carried to them through the interview process. Most had never heard of each other prior to the study. And finally, a number of recommendations are presented in the concluding section relative to how best to innovatively manage innovative people.

One conclusion from this points to the limitations of traditional management models as they are promulgated in the traditional MBA program mold. These were seen everywhere to be counter-productive to the process of environmental improvement. The single focus emphases accounting, marketing, operations, finance, or management and does little to encourage the synthetic attitude environmental issues require. A model for overcoming this is presented under the heading of *virtual management*. Virtual managers are those who do not exist, except for all practical purposes they are managing.

Virtual management is presented as a means to motivate individuals to reach inside a situation instead of being predisposed to listen to the left (public good), or right (private wealth), ear or whatever gets taught in the specific situation of a particular case in a particular management school. This approach is the empirical method of improvement through action learning. It is not the easy empiricism found in case-method. Diagram 1.1 illustrates the emergence of the virtual management method, as it was taken from student drawings of the essentials of management practice. A similar diagram could be made about the parallels between management and regulation methods.

A strict hierarchy is used in model I to accomplish order. In model II a more democratic process is used to bureaucratically manage situations. In model III the individual actor is motivated to find efficient means to achieve a commonly accepted ideal. In model I discussion and consultation are not required. In model II discussion is confined to endless and debilitating committee meetings. In model III a new form of discussion and consultation is critical because the results are implemented.

The optimum model for the ideal manager may prove to be the virtual manager, which is consistent with the most consistently helpful stream that is emerging to replace traditional management theories from Frederick Taylor, et.al. This stream includes what was learned in socio-technical systems management,[52] the Deming

---

[52] This was from the work of Eric Trist, et.al., while at the Tavistock Institute in London during the early 1950s, for the Coal Board of England. What they

approach to quality work, as distinct from quality checkers, and the emergence of autonomous work groups to manage design and product innovation processes.

Some of the technologies outlined in the report were a direct result of the use of this third dimension of management; the negotiated order found in virtual management. One of the most exciting environmental responses found is one that returns to the redesign the total life space of activities and arrives as a very different set of approaches to energy and material uses in the products that support this improved life-space. It comes from designers operating in a management environment like the third model illustrated above. Its results illustrate why pollution filters are intrinsically inefficient, and often counterproductive, how activities like recycling end up being feel-good substitutes for real progress, and why humans need to look elsewhere for more significant and meaningful alternatives.

---

learned is that with complex technologies you cannot design social systems and technical systems in isolation from each other, and you cannot effectively train people to be specialists in managing either one side or the other.

Three Modes of Management

Hard Management for Soft Times, Soft Management for Hard Times

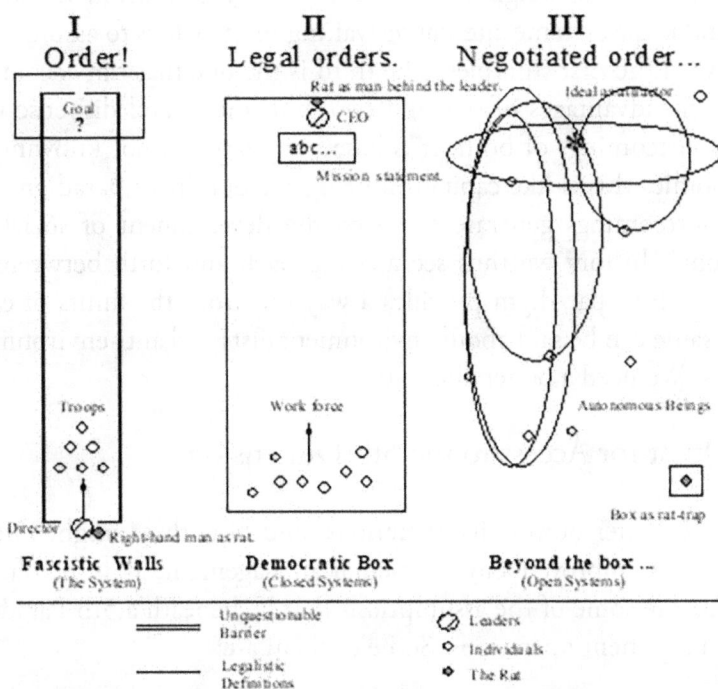

I Order!	II Legal orders.	III Negotiated order...
Goal ?	Rat as man behind the leader. CEO abc... Mission statement	Ideal coordinator
Troops ◇ ◇◇ ◇◇◇	Work force	Autonomous Beings
Director ◇◇ Right-hand man as rat		Box as rat-trap
Fascistic Walls (The System)	**Democratic Box** (Closed Systems)	**Beyond the box...** (Open Systems)

Unquestionable Barrier — Legalistic Definitions

◇ Leaders ◇ Individuals ◆ The Rat

As environmental parties and interest groups become ever more focused, intolerant, and narrow-minded in their outlook, and thus lose their influence in Europe and America it is time to look for how some of their early causes can be realized. One place to look is in Japan, where such parties and groups never have had power, yet environmental concerns within the individual citizen remained at a high level. Much learning could take place in this regard under current considerations of what is sustainable development. In the best sense the core question is: Do current economic actions shortchange the possibilities of our children's well-being? This is a mobilizing concern. During the past fifty years the dominant individual conceptualization has shifted from concern for: "How best might we inherent the earth from our fathers, to how best can we respond to having borrowed it from our children?" This question sounds increasingly like a doorway into the elusive 3rd paradigm that eventually surfaces in public policy discussions.

The first paradigm is always the dominant model in action, the second is the extreme alternative waiting in the wings to assume control with the first stumbles. The third is the one that can accommodate the advantages of one and two, plus more, and dispense with the shortcomings of both. It is based on learning, not knowing. In economics this is like capitalism being the dominant paradigm, but its shortcomings generate and feed the development of socialism. Through history we thus see a swing back and forth between the two. A third paradigm provides a way out from the limits of each. The same can be said about environmentalists and anti-environmentalists. We need a better alternative.

2. Quest for Access to the 5th Dimension

To better outline its operations, and how these might inform and assist improved environmental management, it is helpful to investigate some of the assumptions that lie beneath a 5th Paradigm of management operations. Some of them are:

1. Isms limit the road to substantive improvement. Capitalism and environmentalism both offer limiting visions. Tolerance of other attitudes and approaches, e.g., those seen in both 1st and 2nd paradigms, is essential to the 3rd paradigm appreciation.

2. Choice of dichotomies becomes one of the most important decisions we can make. The traditional differences between long-term and short-term, small, and large, and theory and practice are not helpful to the situation we now face. We need to instead find differences that can make a difference.

3. That placing faith in hi-technology or low-technology is a false dichotomy. Looking into other dimensions of technol-

ogy, such as progress towards the virtual technology ideal of miniaturization, can be more beneficial. This is where the most sophisticated technology is that which becomes smaller in essence and effect until it isn't there, except for all practical purposes it performs.

4. That technology development always outpaces regulation efforts and thus regulation processes become feedback that always misses the target because it has always moved by the time the agent arrives.

5. That governmental regulation has always operated best via acceptance of the ideal hidden in its contract with the body politic that supports it - an organization governs best that governs least.

6. That organizational management operates best that organizes a situation where little is needed to be done - the most successful manager is the one that is not needed.

7. That each person out to do the best for themselves ends up, indirectly, doing the best for society be turned upside down so that each person out to do the best for society ends up doing the best for themselves.

In addition, there is a set of guidelines that come from and fit within the above assumptions. Three, for Environmental Management, are:

1. Each manager operate so as to distribute responsibility for that which turns out well and accept responsibility for that which turns out badly.

2. Each person has a repertoire of behaviors, including some that are highly competitive and some that are very collaborative. Competition works best if it is directed against

ignorance in self and others, not against the nationality, personality, race, sex, or any distinguishing traits of others. Collaboration, on the other hand, works best in response to an impending threat.

3.   The ideal manager is like the ideal regulator, she operates in a way that eliminates the need for her role.

In the following is work from that 1975-77 study. It came from the very serious involvement of industry/government leadership in order to compare company practices from their operating in several countries, and under varied approaches to regulation. The study was to gain insight into the practices and consequences of governance schemes set up for environmental protection. Early on it was noted that there were fundamental differences in how relations to the environmental were governed in Sweden and the United States. This basis was then used to gauge the intentions, operations, and consequences of the two extremes in regulation. A collection of companies were selected as the information base. The total set included all the industrial firms with production facilities in both Sweden and the US. The emphasis was with the plant managers, and those responsible for promulgating and enforcing the environmental laws that governed the facilities.[53] The comparative sets were selected via similarity of inputs, outputs, products, processes, ownership, and management systems. This allowed for control of many of the traditional industrial variables of environmental protection, thus the focus could be with government's role and its relative effectiveness.

---

[53] The study began with twenty company participants in six countries. In a few months the national approaches were reduced to the two of greatest difference. The companies were reduced to the ten with most similar production facilities in both countries . Thus Sweden and the US became the focus of learning. Additional facilities, from the same companies in other countries were visited and examined. Some of these had significant differences in pollution control potentials, such as one redesigned and rebuilt five times to produce English alloys.

3. A Two-Year Project on Regulating Environmental Deterioration

David L. Hawk, Visiting Researcher
Stockholm School of Economics
Institute of International Business

ABSTRACT

The report, *Environmental Protection: Analytic Solutions in Search of Synthetic Problems: Volumes 1-3,* offered a general framework for environmental review. The central difference in method and results is the between the analytic and synthetic. It is used as a standard to compare different methods for governing the relations between human actions and the living systems that make up the natural environment. The emphasis of the analytic is reduction of function. The emphasis of synthetic is composition of activities. Dilemmas exist in both approaches, but the most serious questions arise from the consequences of the analytic. Any argument is presented relative to how the analytic method is at the root of many problems humans have with their larger environment. As such, it is difficult to envision how analysis can be successful in structuring a solution to a problem generated by its method.

The Swedish facilities were consistently cleaner than those in the US. Both had deficiencies in meeting the long-term needs of growing paradoxes, dilemmas, and contradictions behind and in environmental deterioration from human activities. The governance systems of both countries leaned on scientific shortcomings and regulatory optimism. Lawyers, political scientists, and economists in both nations gave too much credit to the knowledge capabilities of the natural sciences.

The predominate paradigm of science used in environmental production relied on problem-solving through dissection, segmentation, and partial analysis to divide the large complex problems into "manageable packages." This is widely known as the science of reductionism. It is the essence of the thought process that had allowed

separation between action and consequence, which had created pollution problems in the first place. A different approach was seen to
be essential. Environmental phenomena had become increasingly
complex and counter intuitive. Use of traditional analytic packaging
systems appeared to as a way to manage through creating manageable
parts. The results illustrate that this form of conventional wisdom is
insufficient to the needs of environmental regulation. Alternatives
are needed.[54] Study participants agreed that to ignore the need for
such and continue with business as usual would encourage conditions to be known as climate change consequences.

The Swedish to corporate and governmental governance
encouraged human adaptation and self-correction at the most local
levels of government and companies. This was where the impacts of
the problems could be most easily felt and quickly responded to. The
approach came to be called "appreciative regulation." The process of
arriving at it and maintaining it was called a "negotiated order."

The US approach was interesting because of its insistence on
centralization of the knowledge-creating, law-making and enforcement processes. It was based on use of legal precision to bring confrontational behavior against the pollution enemy.[55] Those at the
most local levels were considered obstructions and lacking in the
knowledge base required for adequate responses. Even the corporations were skeptical of their local (plant) level management systems.
System inconsistencies, when encountered in carrying out the plans,
tended to bring anger and counter-productive behavior into industry
and government interactions. The US approach is described as legalistic regulation set up to instill a system of legal order.

It is projected that the US environmental management system
will require significant restructuring. During the next 25 years the
US can expect to pass through stages of: tough regulation, de-regula-

---

[54] Concurrent research illustrated that as much as 95% of the environmental
research sponsored to make policy decisions had unfortunately come back after
an irreversible decision had already been taken.

[55] The US tradition seemed to be to let things go for as long as possible, then
declare war on them, invest large sums of money, and then walk away when the
issue is not resolved.

tion, anti-regulation, non-regulation and once again return to tough regulation.

Changes are at this time being considered for the Swedish system. They will probably be consistent with the findings of a Parliamentary Commission established to make regulation more robust in the face of emerging environmental paradox and change, and a need to have more efficient regulations. The Swedes are considering a plan to become more adaptive through becoming more decentralized.

Facility measurements suggest that the Swedish approach is somehow more successful in reducing pollution than the US system. Swedish facilities achieved lower levels of effluent emission than did their US counterparts. Most participants were surprised by the results. Participants felt that, at least in the short term, the US facilities should be and would be cleaner. They were perceived to be surrounded with tough, precise limits, which everyone had to meet. With extensive advice on best available technology from the regulators the US facilities were assumed to be cleaner. Swedish facilities, on the other hand, faced ambiguous limits, little coercion, and company management was given a government request to reduce pollution as much as possible. The most used phrase was "We have a problem, and we would like your help in solving it. We are not sure what to do."

The softer approach to government involvement had somehow ended up achieving higher levels of problem appreciation and lower levels of pollution.[56] Upon reflection, participants felt that Sweden's bias towards cooperation between companies, government agencies, and citizen groups appeared to instill a more inventive and innovative basis for new technologies and their efficient management. This is also seen to be a strong base for future discussions of genuinely effective future processes for reduction of pollution, and not just the continued management of consequences of inefficiency. In addition,

---

[56] In Sweden all the companies in an industry were gathered into a room and were essential told that: "We have a problem. We would appreciate your help. Do the best you can." In the US anti-trust regulations kept industry groups from meeting and a highly competitive value system kept them from working together even if an EPA representative was present.

the Swedish system emphasizes being comprehensively simple.[57] All environmental laws were contained on 25 pages. Their system also encourages inter-institutional experiments in future opportunities.

The US system, designed in a manner consistent with its constitution, was designed to discover truths via battles between governmental agencies, against industry, and between citizens and everything. The model was Platonic in that it sought truth via conflict with a philosopher king regulating the limits. Also in the Greek tradition the confrontation came from the analytic separation of pollution sources and problems. With time they were divided into increasingly narrow streams with conflict in between the streams. Legalistic details were drawn up to attempt resolution of questions prior to their happening, and to avoid exceptions at all costs. Unfortunately, the uncertainties, complex paradoxes[58] and numerous contingencies ended up having to be tried in courts or accommodated outside the law in private anger and with freedom from individual responsibility[59].

The conclusions show that the US regime was organized around the ideal of imposing an order through strictly enforced laws that would coerce people to do what they were not prepared to do. This method was effective in raising the lowest points of environmental response, those who refused to do anything, but over the long term

---

[57] The entire set of environmental laws were written on twenty-five pages. When contrasted to the US highly legalistic system of tens of thousands of pages of laws and directives the Swedes countered that "We feel a pre-condition to citizens obeying the law is to understand it."

[58] US citizens were seen to want increasing protection from the consequences of their actions by the governments they elect, but also demand freedom from governmental interference in their activities. US citizens want more regulation and less control, and for others to solve the problems that they couldn't possibly have created. Politicians are expected to solve the inconsistencies. Many in the study felt these characteristics showed that US citizens were not serious about environmental problems or solutions.

[59] The antidotal stories of how individuals got even with the system were numerous and worrisome. In some regions the Mafia provided an alternative pollution control regime.

it tended punish and lower the high points by discouraging enthusiastic technical innovations.

In addition, the US system was built upon a series of contradictions. It was highly coercive, but it could not, and would not, interfere with the internal operations and confidentiality of business management. The body politic of the US system is filled with contradictions about its support of environmental protection regulation as well. People would demand strong government actions, to manage pollution, but they didn't want the actions to cost them anything, or to modify their lifestyle. In addition, many Americans have come to feel that the Environmental Protection Agency, and their government, is ultimately more responsible for solving environmental problems than are the citizens who create the problems.

Swedish emphasis begins with a low-profile governmental approach to environmental issues. Here industrial collaboration and cooperation between industry and government is used to get participants to first appreciate that there is a serious problem, and then to motivate their joint working towards the yet to be defined solutions. The best ideas for environmental solutions were found to lie with the industry labs and production facilities. It was suggested that they needed to be encouraged and even given incentives to eagerly participate and experiment. The Swedish environmental regime goes to the edge of general discussions of how to limit pollution instead of just how to manage the results of it not being limited.

The regimes of both countries were seen to fall short by tending to generate a growing number of pieces with little idea of how to fit them together again.[60] This happens via the sanctity of analysis and specialization as a religious order. Few people have an idea that the pieces must somehow fit into a whole. The use of legalistic language and process, and coercive behavior, was found to only worsen the situation. This is the same as the industrial model that created the products that end up with the pollution streams in question.

---

[60] This was seen in the proliferation of sub-problems of environment: air, water, solid, toxic, workers, homes, transport, wilderness, etc. This allowed environment to become a packaging problem.

An alternative approach is needed for industry and government in both countries. Herein it is called the appreciative approach. It is non-formal and based on negotiation behavior. Its enemy is the arrogance of those who "know," especially when they have very limited knowledge.[61] The resulting process is a "negotiated order" that accommodates the linkages between human concerns, facts and values, and the need for environmental concern based on values and well as facts as part of an enlarged human experience. One approach suggested by participants to achieve this is to expand the environmental focus to include issues of energy use and economics efficiency into a larger whole. Participants pointed out how the separated activities in each of the three tend to undo gains made in the others.

The Swedish system contained many of the desirable characteristics mentioned above yet they were not yet organized into a coherent framework. As the discussion moves from large scale environmental pollution management to pollution reduction[62] a framework can be expected to appear. More about these summary conclusions can be seen in the three volumes.

Volume I: Environmental Review: Analysis

> This section outlines the general theory of environmental review and protection. The shortcomings of environmental impact assessment and the limitations of reductionistic versions of science are outlined. The Swedish and US approaches to environmental regulation are also presented.

---

[61] There was a great amount of second-rate science in the area of environmental regulation. This was where scientific interpretation, with limited data, was used as a means to justify the ends.

[62] Carl Gerstacker, Chairman of Dow Chemical Co. had addressed the subject via: "Management's Role in Pollution Control." A later speech on "Profits and Pollution" went into more detail on how pollution control could be a source of profit as well as a means for good corporate citizenship: a) sharing knowledge on pollution control, b) reducing waste at the source, and c) enlisting the help of every employee. Until the early 1970's Dow was on the road to an environmental policy that would lead to significant waste reduction. As Washington became increasingly confrontational Dow dropped many of its plans.

Volume II: Environmental Review in Operation: A Need for Synthesis

> This section contains the case material for the study. The results from the twenty facilities that were monitored are presented. The section concludes with a comparative presentation of the structure of the two different national regulatory regimes.

Volume III: Learning from Environmental Review: Seeking Synthesis

Based on the information presented in the first two sections this section moves into the argument that there is a need for synthesis, for new paradigms of environmental understanding and management, and for shifting the ultimate responsibility for environmental issues back towards the individual units of society.

It was thus responded: Governments lack sufficient resources and flexibility to adequately respond to analysis, let alone seeking synthesis. Various reports were made in the media of the 1975-77 research project. They mostly focused on the change in the companies that took place via the research results, prior to the boards of those same companies resorting back to business as usual in the oil and chemical industries. Reports in the Guardian were typical of this:

By the mid-1970's, the biggest oil company in the world, Exxon, was starting to wonder if climate change might finally be about to arrive on the political agenda and start messing with its business model. Maybe it was the reference in the Kissinger speech, or Schneider's appearance on the Tonight Show. Or maybe it was just that the year 2000 – the point after which scientists warned things were going to start to hurt – didn't seem quite so far off.

> In the summer of 1977, James Black, one of the top science advisors at Exxon, made a presentation on the greenhouse effect to the company's most senior staff along with David

Hawk. This was a big deal: executives at that level would only want to know about science that would affect the bottom line. The same year, the company hired Edward David, Jr to head up their research labs. He had learned about climate change while working as an advisor to Nixon. Under David, Exxon started to build a small research project on carbon dioxide. Small, at least, by Exxon standards – at $1m a year, it was a good chunk of cash, just not much compared with the $300m a year the company spent on research at large. He was late to join a project organized in Sweden by David Hawk of the Stockholm School of Economics. Hawk's final report outlined the probability for climate change if humans could not change their behavior. The report by David Hawk came from his project, *Environmental Protection: Analytic Solutions in Search of Synthetic Problems.* It was the founding project of IIB, Stockholm School of Economics, begun in 1975.

In December 1978, Henry Shaw, the scientist leading Exxon's carbon dioxide research, wrote in a letter to David that Exxon "must develop a credible scientific team" one that can critically evaluate science that comes in on the topic, and "be able to carry bad news, if any, to the corporation". (Alice Bell, July 5, 2021, *Guardian News, London.*)

Since 1977 two additional reports have been written at the Wharton School of Finance. The first was titled: *Regulation of Environmental Deterioration*, Philadelphia, Pa.:*S³ Notes Publications*, The Wharton School at the University of Pennsylvania, 1979. Since 1979 an unpublished[63] book chapter was written, titled as "Regulation of the Non-Rational."

---

[63] The editor, Eric Trist, went into the hospital for surgery during the editing process and passed away from us. We continue to miss him. A copy of the chapter can be obtained from the author.

4. Changing the Research Assumptions

> To change our thinking from looking backwards for the "causes" of "effects" to the future to see the greater danger in further effects from the prior effects. (David Hawk, for an OECD Lecture)

Having never appreciated the approach of seeking the cause of an effect as it then led you deeper and deeper towards the irrelevance of nothingness. I would instead look the opposite direction from effects causes to future effects from the current effects as they unraveled. Ambrose Bierce clearly presented the limitation of cause-effect analysis in 1882:

> "Effect, n. The second of two phenomena which always occur together in the same order. The first, called a Cause, is said to generate the other – which is no more sensible than it would be for one who has never seen a dog except in pursuit of a rabbit to declare the rabbit the cause of the dog." [64]

Thus, I came to appreciate the systemic behavior of effects from effects. This was well articulated by Hasan Ozbekhan in his arguing for humans to move attention from problems to problematiques; from abstraction is what isn't to understanding interwoven systems of interconnected problems. As such we need to see "light" not parts as parts of parts, each seeking to be the most important. Use of such thinking ensures the future is more problematic than the now. Via the information from partial analysis, we only ensure great productivity in doing the wrong things wrongly.

In July 1980 Carl Sagan and David Hawk presented ideas in a joint session at the "First Global Conference on the Future," in Toronto, Canada. Conference managers organized it as a combined session of Sagan's forthcoming Cosmos and Hawks completed proj-

---

[64] Ambrose Bierce, The Devil's Dictionary, New York: Hill and Wang, 1957, p 42

ect on Environmental Deterioration leading to climate change. Both presentations addressed the seeming absence of critical faculties to find a way through and forward from mental hopelessness.

> "Far beyond the organizers' expectations, this widely adver-
> tised event attracted some 5,000 registrants. .... Whether
> directly or indirectly, many of the sessions focused on issues
> of environment, natural resources, and conservation. The
> Opening Plenary ranged from a group of neo-Malthusians
> – notably Lester Brown, or the World-watch Institute,
> Aurelio Peccei, of the Club of Rome, and economist Hazel
> Henderson – against a group of cornucopian optimists led
> by Herman Kahn. The first group anticipates that grow-
> ing human numbers and growing human aspirations will
> impose ever-greater pressures on our natural resource-
> base, until ecological backlash and laws of thermodynam-
> ics require an adjustment of human communities to the
> Biosphere's carrying capacity. By contrast, the optimists
> assert that we have hardly started to exploit the most abun-
> dant and renewable resource of all, namely ingenuity as
> expressed through technological know-how."[65]

Sagan and Hawk addressed concerns that humans were operating in limits set by the entropic process, not by human ingenuity and imagination for overriding entropy. Hawk presented the results of his study from 1975-77 that included twenty companies and six governments to see if it was possible to control the human drift towards global climate change via more focused regulation on other humans. Sagan outlined his forthcoming TV show series on "Cosmos." 15 years later, in 1995 Carl Sagan summarized his 1980 concerns about the human condition in one of his books. Therein he wrote:

---

[65] *Abstract of the Conference of 1980*, Norman Myers, Senior Associate of World Wildlife Fund, Cambridge University Press, Aug 24, 2009.

I have a foreboding of an America in my children's or grandchildren's time — when the United States is a service and information economy; when nearly all the key manufacturing industries have slipped away to other countries; when awesome technological powers are in the hands of a very few, and no one representing the public interest can even grasp the issues; when the people have lost the ability to set their own agendas or knowledgeably question those in authority; when, clutching our crystals and nervously consulting our horoscopes, our critical faculties in decline, unable to distinguish between what feels good and what's true, we slide, almost without noticing, back into superstition and darkness.[66]

"Environmental review" was a term specifically defined for the research to serve as an ideal and a focus for the research interviews. It was used as a generic concept for a process of raising questions for social debate about the possible impacts of man's actions on the environment of that action. A concept in common use at the time of the beginning of the research - environmental assessment — served as a basis for development of the ideal concept before an ideal was found necessary. One objective important to environmental review was social debate, where the research discovered that environmental assessment tended to reduce social debate. The importance of social debate for the issues involved in environmental review is seen by looking at the broad spectrum of human activity involved. Utilitarian activities of building highways and factories were found to normally conflict with qualitative domains of beautiful scenery, low noise levels, and interpersonal relations. Past, present, and prospective social value systems as well, are normally brought into such debate. Allowing such a wide spectrum into a review process poses serious problems for the use of strict reductionistic analysis of environmental assessment. Comparing environmental review with the traditional

---

[66] Carl Sagan, The Demon-Haunted World: Science as a Candle in the Dark, New York: Ballantine Books, 1996.

practice of environmental assessment pointed out these and other difficulties with current social mechanisms of problem control, i.e., regulation. The environmental assessment concept was linguistically initiated with the passage of the 1969 National Environmental Policy Act in the United States.

> This Act was the basic mandate to institutionalize environmental considerations into the governmental decision—making process. One of the most noticed aspects of this Act was the process resulting in documents titled "Environmental Impact Statements," or EISs. This Act is important simply due to its existence. It represents a first attempt by a government to formally declare measures for putting environmental concerns into normal decision—making systems.[67]

An argument is posed in the 1977 Report (see pages 8 to 12), that environmental assessment is not conceptually different from the technology assessment of the previous decade but that institutionally they have become very different things. One concern initiating the research, and motivating its continuation was information that most members of the Western industrialized world were looking to the U.S. version of environmental assessment to duplicate versions of it in their own nation's regulatory systems. Members of the OECD (Organization for Economic Cooperation and Development) exemplified this.

Part I of The 1977 Report presented the argument behind environmental review, dominant concepts and practices in current accepted use, and an outline of the major regulatory components required for its operation in Sweden and the United States. Also, Part I examines the role of government as the main initiator of the review activity. As the research was based on comparing Swedish and U.S. regulation systems, relevant statutes and agencies of the respective nations were listed In Part I. A portion of the considerable descriptive

---

[67] The 1977 Report, p. 39

complexity involved in environmental assessment, as it is now practiced, is exposed in Part I. This helps in the later discussion of the
contradictions resulting from complexity.

In Part Il the focus shifts from components of environmental
review of the operations and their consequences of environmental
review. While government was the major actor in Part I, industrial
production facilities are the emphasis in Part 11. Characteristics of
each industrial type represented in the research are presented as well
as specifics of cases researched. Basic to the examination of the cases
are the "legal permits" required to operate the facilities within allow-
able levels of pollution. The models, methods, and basic concepts
relied on to gain and structure information were presented in Part II.
This provided a basis for discussing some of the dilemmas of current
environmental assessment operations.

Combining the governmental social system sets described in
Part I with the industrial sets described in Part 11 allows a view of
the complexity involved in the regulation of environmental affairs
and offers a base to examine the failures of current regulatory systems
attempting to control the complexity. (This was especially so within
the U.S. context.)

In Part III the theoretical development for an alternative to
the existing modes of environmental protection regulation is begun.
In this part an idea of Hasan Ozbekhan (1974) was espoused (that
complex problems which society is faced with are not problems in
the traditional sense of the word). A "problem" cannot be assumed
to be something which has a "solution." Instead, we can think in
terms of situations. Ozbekhan's ideas give additional support to the
thesis repeatedly put forward here, that we cannot treat the complex
situations we are faced with as if they are problems merely waiting
for the proper solution to arrive after rigorous analysis. Some of the
systems logic of Emery (1969) and Ackoff (1974) is presented in Part
III to serve as a basis for an alternative paradigm for dealing with
complex societal situations, where the environmental protection situation is one example. This alternative logic is coming to be known
as "Systems Thinking" (Emery, 1969). The following is a summary
of current attempts to "improve" the environment by protecting it.

This research concludes that the environmental protection effort will not satisfy the needs behind the concern for an individual's environment and its quality. Although the need to question the trend of technical manifestations of current social thinking was legitimate, we have only furthered specialization and have lost the composite social understanding of current efforts to question technology. Lack of composite understanding in a society manifests itself in fear of the unknown. Through an elaborate analytically technical approach we have advanced two wrongs: 1) Through the use of the word "protection" we have introduced a negative connotation, which adds to fear, 2) And by turning the environmental issue over to the experts we have seen it dissected and parceled out in a manner that further obscures whatever holistic meaning it may have once had.[68]

5. Research Results

Chapter 5 outlines key information with future significance for long—range environmental protection activities. The information in this chapter was directed at short—term circumstantial evidence relating to immediately discernable results. In this summary an attempt is made to link these two varieties of data together. Even the more circumstantial evidence implies longer-range consequences when given understandable structure.

The discussion in Chapter 2 on two modes of regulation, formal legislative and informally negotiated, specified the characteristics of the two modes. Some of this information clarifies the research data. One means of comparing the alternative modes is to weigh the research data against the modes by following the role of facts, in each of the cases. (Facts relate to those things "known to be true.") Within the framework of the "legal order" approach deliberated actions are generally taken by a group of experts competent at getting into the

---

[68] Hawk, 1977, p. 193

"facts of the case"; at least such is an ideal as expressed by those hiring the experts. There also is an assumption here that facts have a relatively long lifespan. Also, they generally are oriented towards the technical domains of the situation. Factors associated with human variables, like interpersonal relations, are not included, whenever possible. The "negotiated order" mode, on the other hand, is based on development of the appreciation systems which underlie the ordering of facts. Here the facts of the case take on a role of reduced consequence, due to the considerable uncertainty present in the situation allowing facts to fluctuate with perceptions of the situation. When the facts become ambiguous, even contradictory, the behavioral factors can explicitly play a larger role in decisions. Interpersonal relations can then be openly relied on to mutually define an ambiguous situation, or to redefine a mutually objectionable situation. Under a legal order system this is implicit; with a negotiated order it becomes explicit. Under legal order, facts become an end in themselves; with negotiated order facts and values are part of a larger process giving normative direction to both. The information in the cases is now related to the two alternatives of regulation.

1. Location of Responsibility (in terms of a center—periphery model of control)
2. Regulation Modes Impacting on Large versus Small Organizations
3. Growing Interdependencies of Industry and Industrial Process and Growing Fragmentation of the Regulation Processes
4. Trust versus Surveillance as an Attitude

Here it has been seen that most of the issues intertwined with the environmental objectives of material pollution control are highly social—behavioristic concerns. Even in the few cases where the "facts of the case" are relatively clear, very little occurs in a positive direction until human behavior allows it. It is important that there be a joint recognition that changes need to be instituted and then joint design of those changes. An appreciation of each other's point of departure and point of view in a situation is helpful to resolution of problems in a situation.

Although many of the results of the case studies appeared rather diverse, they did tend to settle into the interpersonal realm, at least indirectly. For all individuals the initial attitude that dominated was to discover the problem, find its cause and then offer a resolution. This was soon seen to lead to additional problems since cause-effect models missed the systemic behavior of the whole. Once this was seen those involved stepped back and adopted three attitudes found to arrive at better, more systemic, results. They were a choice between 1) cooperation, 2) confrontation, and then movement on to 3) a mixture of 1 and 2, then ending in mostly 1) from worry for the difficulty of the problems.

These could also be considered strategies, but they seemed to cover more than consciously planned activities; in fact, they tended to permeate the individual's personality. Besides cooperation and confrontation, the mixed area formed a vast gray area where individuals appeared uncommitted to either. Instead, they appeared to be trying to get hold of the situation they were in by slowing it down so they could understand it. Perhaps the concept of Donald Schon (1971) called "dynamic conservatism" best labels this group. For purposes of classifying the interviewees, this group was termed "the baffled." The dominant characteristic of those who tended to rely on cooperation was that they tended to "compose" the elements of a situation, while those relying on confrontation "analyzed" a situation for resolution.

Based on careful review of review of the ten companies involved in the final version of the study and those involved in the final twenty cases in the study. Each company had a refinery or factory in both of the two nations we came to focus on. Therein we documented an array of successes and failures of pollution control or management.

Thus, we have the following three types of leaders:

Type I   The "Expert Analyzer" relying on subdivisions of wholes into ever more partial parts in order to become Confrontational. For him the idea of solving effects is to locate the cause; that there are no causes to what matters is simply irrelevant. Trust is not relevant; context is noisy; if there is a problem there must be a solution. Find it.

Type II   Committee Member Type as a Silent Watcher, essentially "The Baffled." Committees are primarily established to keep an eye on those that should not be trusted, i.e., others. Passive acceptance of complexity in environments and others is okay; especially if it not understood by the committee.

Type III   Cooperative Personality, as "The Composer." This is the type who sees relationships between parts (as connections), not parts floating in isolation. Such a person works to synthesize all elements. to reduce appearance of complexity as traditionally created by humans to hide what they wish to avoid. The Composer trusts everyone, especially the untrustworthy as it destabilizes their strategy. Crucial to cooperation is learning. This person never takes critic for what goes well, but quickly picks up the blame for what is seen as a bad idea.

ATTITUDE TYPOLOGIES OF LEADERS OF PROJECTS

An apparent difference existed in the attitudes in Sweden versus those seen in the U.S. This came to be clarified in a seminar offered at the Stockholm School of Economics in October of 1976. The purpose of the seminar was for participants of the main organizations in the research to discuss issues raised in the research to that date and advise on future directions of the research. There were twenty—two participants at the seminar, with all but two of the organizations in the research represented. In most cases the representative was the chief executive of the organization, or from top management if not the top executive. It was very interesting to find that such a meeting was possible in Sweden, especially when compared with interview information of similar people in the U.S., which concluded that such a meeting would not be allowed in the U.S. for anti—trust and other behavioral reasons.

The information mentioned previously has been organized in the above composite chart. It's to compare the cooperation/confrontation characteristics with the location of decision—making responsibility and with the results of the permit for each case in the study.

6. Conclusions from the Project

The research conclusions were organized about the areas of management thought at the time to be crucial to operation of environmental protection concern.

a) A theory of regulation

Since this dissertation itself is directed at the development of a theory of regulation there is little value to concentrating on the theory within the 1977 Report. The tenuous theory found there was mainly concerned with the location of regulatory responsibility, where the report bias was towards a decentralized system of regulation which could accommodate the considerable variety in modern society. This dissertation develops a theory of regulation in terms of the holistic operation of a regulation system where the location of the responsibility for control is only one component of the whole.

b) The role of the expert

Centralization of control tends to correlate well with increased reliance on experts, at least within the environmental protection area.

As such any viable theory of regulation must address questions concerning the location and role of the expert in that regulation. The extensive role of the expert throughout the enforcement of regulation has come to be accepted and even expected. Some of the dangers of this phenomenon were pointed out in the 1977 Report, where one example in the U.S. comes out of the Environmental Protection Agency. The regulation of the environment was legislatively divided up into eight major parcels (see Part I of the 1977 Report), but once the enforcement of these parcels began, they were further divided along expert discipline lines. The problem with this is that each discipline developed its own practices and policies. In too many cases there was substantial conflict between either of the two practices and/or policies, where all seemed to be removed from local reality.

In addition, it was discovered within the research that expert decisions were the justification for much of the statute design itself. If there is value in retaining the political processes which Americans feel they have, then this reliance on expert decision—making seems to deny much of that value. In the U.S. Congress there are 435 Representatives, 100 Senators, and 11,000 aides to advise them. As United States society has become more complex the reliance on expert aides to supply decision—making information has greatly increased.

> The problems confronting Congress have become so technical and the problems so complicated that they demand the attention of specialists. A Congressman simultaneously faced with proposals concerning automobile safety, deregulation of natural gas pricing, Federal funds for abortion and the revision of the Panama Canal Treaty would crumble in confusion unless he could rely on expert advisors or committee staff directors...[69]

This does not sound so worrisome, but this trend has generated a power shift that does cause concern; especially so if experts live up to their definition of only having specialized knowledge of a

---

[69] Newsweek, August 15, 1977, p. 27

very limited part of a situation. It appears that the trend of increased reliance on experts in regulation complements the trend of fractionalization of industrial societies.

> With Congress currently more fragmented than it has ever been, the power of legislative aides has soared. Senators and Representatives were found to function more independently rather than collectively. Members of Congress were seen act as virtually autonomous barons and hence more dependent than ever on their professional staffs. The major deviations came from visits with lobbyists that were seen as essential to the standing of the member of Congress. As a result, much of the consequential legislation passed by Congress in recent years has been the work of individual Congressmen, their assistants, and lobbyists rather than the result of Congressional Committees or joint efforts.[70]

The dilemma underlying this is that as the society becomes more interdependent and complex, the mode of regulation is becoming more fractionalized. As well as the legislative branch of the U.S. regulatory system basing its operations on the overreliance on experts, the court system is now having to retain to its own extensive collection of experts. In the research a very workable alternative to expert fractionalization was uncovered in Sweden in what is called the National Franchise Board. (See page 25 of the 1977 Report for further explanation of the design and composition of the Board.) The work of this Board compares well with the principles of "negotiated order" presented in Chapter 2 of this paper.

c) Redefinition of environment

The issues of environmental deterioration and environmental protection are overlaid with negative overtones. Environmental deterioration appears as a very nasty phenomenon but was seen as mostly

---

[70] Ibid.

outside definition. Environmental protection, as a response, implies creating a stand—off, where although the environment may not be improved, at least it will not be allowed to worsen. At the outset of environmental concern in the late 1950's to early 1960's the negative aspects were not such a noticeable issue. Much of this was due to the vague character of the environment where the vagueness allowed flexibility of meaning and direction. (In line with this the vagueness allowed traditionally divergent interests to fit under the same umbrella and work collectively for what was felt to be a common cause.) When environmental issues started to be defined in narrower terms of pollution, and what constituted pollution, the negative connotation began to overpower the initial general environmental ethic. This has serious repercussions for the mechanisms of enforcement of any specific system of regulation. For example,

> If a central authority must play a role in environment — and under current conditions, it cannot withdraw due to the attitudes and dependencies it has built up — the least the authority can do is to coordinate regulation activities in a positive and creative manner. A positive tone to regulation allows for more desirable and voluntary participation of the regulated with the regulators; where the ideal is for the two to merge into one group. Unless society is able and willing to furnish one "policeman" per pollution source, a Teutonic, or totalitarian, system cannot be successful. A system designed to force actions out of one set of people, by another set, which the first are not in logical support of, will only have limited successes. Research shows that "actions" will result from such a system of regulation, but they will not be the most desirable for either party, or the larger society which both parties are a part of.[71]

In many instances' "environment" has been used as a weapon to force individuals to do something they would not want to do.

---

[71] The 1977 Report, p. 198

The difficulty is that force instills fear at best and encourage hate at worst towards the target and the enforcer. Several dimensions of the phenomenon called <u>threats</u> has been presented in a book entitled, <u>The Effects of Threats</u> by George Kent (1967). Even if the concept of force could be handled effectively - which appears in democratic societies that it should not or cannot be - another dilemma awaits a forceful regulation of major social issues. Having the power to force an action does not guarantee one the knowledge of how best to carry it out, or, in essence, "omnipotence does not insure access to omniscience." (Perhaps too great of a concentration on the first may restrict the second.)

d) Utilizing environmental review for "learning"

It Is important to notice the sense of learning used in the 1977 Report, as it underlies the logic of the alternative mode of regulation called negotiated order. The capacity to generate alternatives to deal with a confronted situation is essential to learning. The 1977 Report defined a "non—learning" situation as one where there were no alternatives to deal with it beyond a simple yes or no response to a stimulus. Four types of learning were listed in a hierarchical fashion, from "zero—base" to "learning type III." These were an elaboration of Gregory Bateson's (1973) "learning types." For him "zero base" is simply a "response to a stimulus" and no real choice is available. Learning III on the other hand involves such a wide latitude of possible choices that, if an individual takes this route, he questions the most basic assumptions. This model of learning was used In The 1977 Report to analyze some of the limitations of current environmental review and, illustrate why environmental review choices are so severely limited.

The two arguments for environmental review, or environmental impact assessment, are: 1) it enhances public participation and 2) it generates alternatives. With traditional environmental impact assessment, the research found little evidence of the process enhancing public participation and no evidence that viable alternatives were generated by the process. In fact there was more evidence that the process reduced participation by inducing greater use of experts and specialists. The public is discouraged from taking a "positive" part in the process. Most of the actions they are asked to review are designed in such a manner that the only alternative is between yes or no. This researcher hypothesizes that due to the increasing technical sophistication of future proposed actions, there will be an increasing use of the no alternative as more public participation is elicited. Reasons for this are varied, but two possibilities may be that if you don't understand a proposal you tend to say no for the sake of safety and the chance for this is increased if you can't directly see how the proposal will benefit you and can see how it may harm you.[72]

If learning were an integral part of environmental review, as illustrated in the diagram on page 12 of the 1977 Report, then the review process would be vastly more complex and intellectually difficult. On the other hand, it would have been publicly more credible and have elicited more interest, thereby making it more meaningful and socially desirable. As environmental review is now developing steps are taken to cut back on participation in order that "socially necessary" projects can be approved in a timely fashion. This, of course, further erodes the democratic ideals of the larger society, of which environmental review is only a part.

Throughout the research the role of attitude was emphasized as it appeared to be more important than technology in explaining environmental activities in industry and government. Many of the industrial personnel who worked in both Sweden and the U.S. felt that "The technical innovativeness for environmental protection in the U.S. system is quite high, but the application of the innovation seems to be more successful outside the U.S. Continuing with this feeling.

---

[72] Ibid., p. 199

Our system requires tremendous monitoring. Our office investigates 10% of the major pollution sources in our area each year. This takes 30% of our total manpower resources. It is difficult when you don't trust them.[73]

e) A redirection of attitudes towards environment

The Swedish regulation system is openly more cooperative in its basic attitude towards solving environmental problems than the U.S. system, but a satisfactory resolution of environmental dilemmas will require more than cooperation. This is not to detract from the fact that cooperation as a basis for resolution is essential; but basic knowledge is critical also.

> The difficulty of fighting in all ill—defined complex situation, like environmental deterioration, is that two opponents may well miss each other completely in the darkness or go down the wrong road in parallel.[74]

Beyond the basic value of a cooperative attitude, it is generally important to begin to identify attitudes towards a subject of interest in a problem resolution effort. In the environmental protection area specifically, it is important to identify the dominant attitudes towards the area. This point was alluded to in the section on Redefinition of Environmental Issues[75] where the dominant attitude in the environmental area tends to be, as stated by Rene Dubos:

> It is a sad commentary on our civilization that when we speak of the environment it is usually in reference to its undesirable effects. The very word environment now evokes the nightmares of industrial and urban life, depletion of

---

[73] Ibid., p. 203
[74] Ibid., p. 204
[75] Hawk, 1977, p. 3

natural resources, accumulation of wastes, pollution in all its forms, noise, crowding, regimentation, the thousand devils of the ecological crisis... As a result, we are chiefly concerned with the avoidance of dangers and maintenance of a tolerable state, rather than with the creation of new, positive values through the development of environmental and human potentials.[76]

Dubos has also pointed out the implications of this attitude towards the environment, which in 1978 we can now see realized.

If we limit our efforts to the correction of environmental defects, we shall increasingly behave like hunted beasts taking shelter behind an endless succession of protective devices, each more complex and costly, less dependable, and less comfortable than its predecessors... Although technological fixes have transient usefulness, they complicate life and eventually decrease its quality.[77]

Along with the more positive attitude which believes in human potentialities, there should be a healthy pessimism of outside limitations facing man's endeavors. This is not to restrict man's creativity but to give it an informed direction. In the case of environmental issues, it is important to weigh the available creativity for new solutions to pollution problems with knowledge of the first and second law of thermodynamics.

The first law has great validity in stating that matter can neither be created nor destroyed but this has lured too many with an industrialist interest in mind into believing that there is no material cost associated with using natural resources. These people might well enhance their perception through respect for the second law which notes that although matter may not be created nor destroyed, it does

---

[76] Rene Dubos, 1972, p. 192, as quoted on page 2 of the 1977 Report.
[77] Ibid., p. 1973

go through qualitative changes through use. When a barrel of oil is "burned" it is no longer available for further "burning".

On the other hand, too many with an environmental interest in mind seem to rely on the second law to the exclusion of the limits of the first. They seem to feel that any current use of a material necessarily reduces its quality while at the same time they ask for a "pollution less plant" which means that a great deal of by—product must vanish. Officials in the State of New Jersey typify part of this attitude. The officials noted that there was a significant problem with toxic wastes leeching into groundwater in the state from solid waste disposal sites. They resolved the problem by simply outlawing the disposal of toxic solid waste, with no alternative method of getting rid of it offered. It was then disposed of in less legal ways.

7. Generalizing

The previous information tended to be unique to the cases in the research. Although much of the material was case specific, the collective information body does imply certain things about current modes and manners of regulation. The collective information is presented in terms of general issues, which at a later point are combined to aid in the design of an alternative system of regulation for complex problems.

a) Location of plant management responsibility

Based on the research information it was difficult to ascertain the "best" location of management responsibility for a production facility with major pollution characteristics. In some cases, it was advantageous for major responsibilities to be left with personnel at the facility. In other cases, this proved to be dangerous and counterproductive to environmental goals. In most of the cases it did seem that greater plant autonomy, which means greater responsibilities for decision making at the plant personnel level, was the more desirable approach, especially in terms of technology design and negotiation with government officials. A qualification needs to be made here concerning negotiation; negotiations were considered more successful, in terms of desirable solutions, when both industry and governmental people came from the more "local" level. When central government people were negotiating with plant people, or vice—versa, the outcomes and process were less desirable. As far as the industry aspect was concerned there were two disadvantages to too much involvement in pollution control by headquarters: 1) plant personnel, who were the most involved with day to day operation where most pollution is initiated, felt less responsible or committed to the ideals involved if others took care of negotiations and equipment design, and 2) by depending on a small group of headquarters' staff people for innovation, the opportunities for different approaches were greatly reduced. When a "fixed" solution was applied throughout a company, regardless of contextual factors at the facility, the results were not encouraging.

The dilemma in this issue is that, although more local autonomy may be desirable, the statutes and regulatory agencies are set up in a manner necessitating the use of highly specialized experts during the negotiation process. Since few organizations can afford to have a wide variety of expertise at each facility, the plants rely on headquarters to supply it, or hire consultants through headquarters. This introduces the second major item to emerge from the research data.

b. Difficulties of small businesses dealing with large regulations

Closely associated with the issue of current legislative modes necessitating extensive expert assistance in dealing with regulation activities is the problem of small organizations not having the capacity for this. This problem was initially detected during the research into the smaller firms in the study; and even the "smaller" firms were in the order of one—half billion-dollar gross sales. Based on this initial indication, specific questions were directed at key government officials to see what evidence they had as to how successful small business organizations were in environmental regulation affairs. In addition, some individuals within some small firms (with less than one—hundred million gross sales), were interviewed informally to gain their perceptions on the subject. Many of those interviewed felt their future greatly threatened by increasing levels of regulation; others were not even aware of current legislation which they were obligated to comply with.

A report has been compiled by the Small Business Administration in Washington D.C. which results from a research project into "The Impact on Small Business Concerns of Government Regulations that Force Technological Change." The research investigated regulation in the areas of environmental protection, worker health and safety, and product safety. The report concluded that,

> The impacts of environmental regulations appear greatest on small companies where economies of scale suggest that compliance expenditures per unit of output would be inversely proportional to size, but the surveys reported the smallest companies facing lesser impacts than larger small companies, no doubt a reflection of regulatory exceptions applicable to very small firms... There were also indications that the ratio of compliance spending to total assets is inversely proportional to company size.[78]

Based on evidence gained through interviewing and the SBA Report, the "larger" small industries were spending 20 to 50% of their assets to finance technical modifications. Although the regulation tended to affect smaller industries later than larger industries, this was distinctly not to the small firm's benefit. One reason why a large corporation encountered the regulation sooner was that it had specially trained people working in Washington full time to identify what statutes and policies were emerging before they were finalized. The large corporations could "plan" for potential regulation impacts. The small firms not only could not plan, but they could also not even afford personnel to deal with the regulation activities once regulations began to affect them.

---

[78] SBA Report, 1975

A way of expressing this dilemma which fits into the theme of the development of an alternative mode of regulation follows. Essentially, the governmental regulation system and the large corporations are creating a highly formalized system of planning - not too unlike a long—range comprehensive plan. The small businesses and the more "local" government officials are operating within a more "incremental" planning system that is highly informal and extemporaneous. The formal approach relies on generalizable scientific truths which present the "factos-of-the-case," while behavioral factors are considered secondary. "Facts" are felt to remain the same, regardless of who expressed them; thus, interpersonal relations are not crucial to success. On the other hand, the informal approach relies on inter—personal relations between the main actors to make sense of the facts available. In our situation the first approach — the more formal one - would allow easier regulation. The only argument in favor of the more extemporaneous approach is where there is considerable uncertainty about the facts—of—the—case. The disconcerting feature about environmental protection issues is that the facts are very uncertain, and indeed seem to become more uncertain with time. For example, in the early sixty's government experts felt we could identify the facts involved in environmental quality. A 1975 report by the President's Council for Environmental Quality points out how difficult it now is to determine even the facts of water quality.

> Just as there is no single measure of human health, there is no single measure of water quality. Rather there are dozens of specific physical, chemical, and biological characteristics of the nation's waters.[79]

Currently, there are about sixty quantitative criteria covering forty—three water quality variables for the U.S. Environmental Protection Agency, and the list is growing. In addition, what is considered a "good" measure of one of these variables for one particular

---

[79] CEQ Report, 1975, p. 348

use may in fact be a "bad" measure for another use. See pages 67 to 69 of the 1977 Report for a further discussion of these issues.

If we place social value on retaining smaller social organizations in both public and private sectors — and we do seem to value such — we need an alternative regulation mode for societal problem areas which have considerable uncertainties in them. Even the large social organizations within the research are now finding it increasingly difficult to continue with the highly formalistic approach to regulation which demands high predictability. Perhaps part of the reason why large organizations found the formal method viable at first was due to their initiating costs having gone to smaller organizations, who traditionally were competitors. It now seems that even the competitive ethic has run sour in this type of problem area, the hypothesis being that, under conditions of great uncertainty, competition is harmful to most actors involved and that a more cooperative regulation method is desirable.

c. Production interrelations and regulation separations

Many of the specific issues raised in the cases began to merge, but considered against a context of regulation activities, the issues become separated. Of more immediate significance is a comparison of how interrelated the production aspects of the companies are and how segregated the regulation aspects are. A point which emerged very strongly from the research project was how closely interwoven the companies in the research were. Each production process, each facility, each company, fit into a larger network where the composite formed the industrial system which our current lifestyle depends upon. Even traditional competitors were drawing closer together to deal with the uncertainties of the increasingly complex systems with which they were interacting. Some of the interdependencies were pointed out in the proceedings from a seminar of the major participants in the research held in October of 1976. But, in addition, a chart was put together, with the assistance of individuals from the companies, to illustrate the path which the raw materials pass through on the way to become consumable products. Many firms which were traditionally considered quite separated now have at least a second-ary relationship with each other, if not a primary relationship. For example, a paper production company was beginning to merge with a chemical production company as it was discovered that they were dealing with similar materials and processes but did not have to com-pete for consumers. They had discovered that their longer—range objectives were quite similar, as were their long—range concerns.

The figure on the following page illustrates one dimension of the researched companies' interrelations.

It is especially interesting, from a research standpoint, to note how the differing aspects of the societal industrial process are becom-ing more interlocked while at the regulative systems become increas-ingly fragmented, resulting in that funny smoke screen we call com-plexity, as we embrace its confusion.

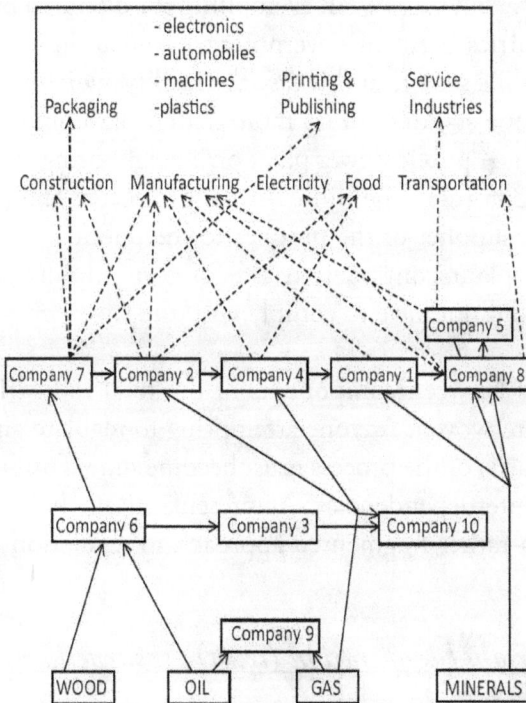

Interdependence of Production

Using Company 9 as an example, the overall company is faced with a wide variety of governmental regulative attempts, in addition to the corporate ones, where Case 9—S was the most holistically regulated facility of the three in the research which this company operates. Two conditions did exist at the Case 9, which stem from characteristics of the plant and its management. One, due to the sensitivity of the plant location, various technical changes were introduced which looked good politically, but which did not match the larger industrial process, nor have they been effective against pollution; and two, where two companies operate the facility, the company from the host country does not add lead to the product while the company from outside the country does.

Case 9-A on the other hand presents almost a worst—case example of fragmented regulation activities. This facility is regulated by three different governmental authorities, each with its own standards and policies. And Case 9—B exemplifies the dilemma building up in many countries between governmental regulation of the private versus the public sector. In this case the facility, which is private, is required to meet a standard of no more than 3% Sulphur content of its final product. A public power plant on a neighboring site is also governed by the 3% rule. The difficulty arises because the plant in the study was the supplier of the product to the public power plant where the power plant continues to ask for 5% Sulphur content, saying, that they did not have to comply with the law.

Connections between components of the total industrial process are closely interwoven. Anyone attempting to regulate any part, or collection of parts, of the process must become more familiar with and respect the interdependencies. At present, in all the countries studied, there is a rather fragmented approach to regulation of production facilities.

d. Interpersonal cooperation (trust) vs. surveillance

A comparison of the actual permits resulting from the regulation activities in Sweden and the U.S. illustrates the consequences of a variation in approaches to policing the targets of a regulation activity and exemplifies how the "trusting" approach becomes more desirable in achieving the objectives of the regulation. Various indications are available within the research of the differences between the more cooperative mode of Sweden and the surveillance mode of the U.S. The basis of the cooperative approach appears to lie in a faith that the members of a given society will, in general, behave in accordance with the best interests of the society of which they are part. This, of course, moves some of the problem focus into the definition of the "best" interests of a society. An advantage of such a move is that if there is agreement that there should be cooperation in identifying "best," at least one element of the "best" is identified. The basis of the close surveillance approach to regulation rests on an assumption that there exist irreconcilable differences of interest between members of a society and that the society, and the members of it must be forced to act in ways that they normally would not. Associated with this is an assumption that the most efficient method of forcing is governmental action from as central as possible.

Based on the research, the Swedish environmental regulation system typifies a more trusting approach while the U.S. regulation attitude relies more on the forcing approach. The following chapter on some of the consequences of different approaches to regulation offers more evidence about the Swedish and U.S. approach to environmental regulation. This information is of a greater degree of generality than that presented in this chapter.

There was no success in applying the findings of very concerned companies and government people forty years ago. They saw an urgent need to control environmental deterioration resulting from human activities. They helped recommend a new model for regulation. The situation was fluid, not fixed, and in need of ideas for business as unusual in both private and public organizations. Back then it was shown how deterioration was expanding and efforts to regulate and limit such were turning bad into worse.

The situation of environmental deterioration can no longer be addressed via expanded research, invention of new technologies or in modifications in meeting humans needs and wants in adjustments to the current neo-classical economic model. We have moved beyond those somewhat understood traditional responses. We now face the consequences of greatly expanded environmental deterioration. It is now culminating in very dire phenomena such as the one only briefly mentioned in the 1977 study called *climate change*. Humans must quickly change. They need to improve business as usual practices in meeting human bio-needs while completely rethinking the holography of their psycho-wants.

Humans need to find responses of a different logical type. The tradition of reductionistic, analytically managed processes in search of cause-effect conclusions, that we are so proud of needs to be abandoned. Positivistic science is not helpful in dealing with systemic reality. The tradition of arrogantly distinguishing humans from nature needs to be left behind. Simply designing tough legislation for stern governance, as based on causal logic, will not lead to success. Stern ignorance only moves success further away, as shown forty years ago in the study reference herein. Deterioration was seen to grow alongside growth in threatening punishment. We should now move from that ideology, not emphasize a value that isn't. Elsewhere, there are signs of optimism, such as in reintroducing longer-term values. Humans learning Consequential Management need to replace MBA educated managers. 19th Century ideas of the greatness of industrialization need to be re-evaluated considering the long-term deterioration harm from short-term economic valuation now appearing.

e) Future Dimensions of Management

A human future requires serious concern for living systems on our planet. We need a way to rethink our past reliance on 2-dimensional regulations, derived via 1-dimensional ideologies from pointless wants for mortal power. We need to look for differences that make a difference. You may say aspects of what follows is complex but keep in mind that accusing something of "being complicated" has long been the excuse to retain business as usual. We now have an urgent need for business as unusual.

The research discussed herein originates fifty years ago. It came from obvious signs of environmental deterioration beginning to have consequential impacts for humans. The actions of humans leading to deterioration had been undertaken in the name of improving human lifestyles. The research showed that humans were not very concerned about the consequences of this choice. They did not what to redefine economic development based on the eternal Faustian Bargain, and its shadow known as the Faustian Tragedy. The logical conclusion of this kind of bargaining with the human future was central to the work of Nicholas Georgescu-Roegen as best represented in his 1971 thesis that current economic models are entropic aids, and end in additional deterioration.

A modified thesis then emerged after several years of research begun in 1975 at the Stockholm School of Economics. It found there to be no viable way to fix neo-classical economics, nor improve traditional governance to slow deterioration of the natural environment. We, my friend Gunnar Hedlund, and I, then proposed a move to "business as unusual" based on developing a non-Faustian economics model. Attempts were made to test this in economic and social development, all in line with expanded appreciation of life's context – nature. The model was to show examples of rejecting human subservient to the ideal of the artificial. To date, the success in this effort has been minimal. Gunnar's 1996 death from a chemically initiated brain tumor was then treated with radiation to fix the problem. After his death the surgeon published a paper on how radiation fixed the cancer problem. Unfortunately, it "fixed" the patient as well. The world of the artificial and its expansion continued.

The central issue forty years ago was the deterioration consequences from an economic model that made dollars, but little sense. The model politically justified a model of production and consumption activities, one that made even less sense to life's continuance than its economic end. The model focused on expansion of the idea of industrialization production and then product use; all presuming eventual regulation of its harmful-to-life consequences.

The study began with concern for industrialized consequences to nature in light of a nineteen-sixties acceptance that environmental

deterioration was the price of life. Those in the study were looking for more effective ways of regulation, to manage the undesirable
from producing the desired. Economists in the study argued that the
contemporary model would adjust to resolve the problem. A group
now known as "ecological economists" argued for going much further with regulation via price manipulations.

A friend and mentor, Nicholas Georgescu-Roegen, argued
against that title, pointing out ecology would consume economics. I
agreed with him, yet the ecological economy greatly expanded in the
next thirty years. So too has environmental deterioration. Perhaps
something deeper is at work; something that relates to nature, each
other, and us? Just now I'm much less optimistic about finding a way
out from the prognosis of our decline. Ecological economics seems
more like another pacifier, in the same class as the pattern of purposeful recycling. We take our trash to the curb. It goes away from
our view. It is not seen again, except in trash dumps or floating in the
oceans. We seem to invest little in experimenting with radical recipes
of business as unusual, a location where schools and enterprises need
to go.

Late in the study, with the collaboration of major Petro-
chemical leaders and scientists, the notion of a phenomenon called
climate change was emerging. This was said to take humans to a fateful end far quicker than anything with environmental deterioration
effects known in prior science. It was posed as a determinant of the
human fate, just as it had been posed in 1858 by the American scientist Eunice Foote, then expanded on by Nobel Laurate Arrhenius
of Sweden. Climate change was seen to be the consequence of continuation of industrialization. The evidence for human creation of
climate change consequences has greatly expanded since. The obvious question then turns to how far have humans come in developing
alternatives to business as usual? What should business as unusual
look like, then how can we encourage it realization? Business as
usual, with its consequences in deterioration is clear. Why do we stay
with business as usual?

It is important to step back and remind ourselves that we have
long had an underlying dilemma behind our ideal of human prosper-

ity. Any projection of industrial consequences from economic thinking, via business as usual, seems bleak. Research from forty years ago
suggested that the consequences will be very dire of failure. It also
demonstrated how the usual approach to regulating problems would
not work. Since then, that fear has become reality. A new model of
regulation is now needed or a new definition of social civilization. The
argument about shortfalls in regulation of environmental deterioration is informative to our current challenge. If nothing else, it seems
to serve as a benchmark of man-nature relations, to see what progress
has been made in appreciating that relation, or not. Comparing the
conversations from "now" to the research "then" allows some understanding of the conditions of life, and their prospects.

More now sense the human situation as becoming dire. Some
progress has been made to improve understanding of the situation,
but not in improving it. If worsening, do we at least understand why
and what needs to be done? For four decades did we at least come to
learn the role of humans in being problematic, and what they need
to change? Can we respond to "what now?"

That seventies study found that traditional regulation was not
working, and possibly could never work. It did find small signs of
hope in non-hierarchical management of the network form. With
some humor this came to be known in the project as a "more anarchistic"[80] version of "human regulation." It somehow operated to
bring out more innovative, more non-rational, repairs to a situation
via what came to be a negotiated order. It was far more interesting
and much more successful than the reliance of the false success in the
rationality of legal order methods. Thus, it seems important that we
review ideas from the research of 1975-1977 to better regulate environmental deterioration.

The strength of negotiated order was seen in the appreciation
it required. The weakness of the legal order was seen in the hollow threats it depended upon but could seldom deliver. Now that

---

[80] This was of the Kropotkin, i.e., Socratic and Lao Tzu, form of anarchism as self-
governance of human-generated problems that mattered most. These tended
to be too much a part of being human to be handled via legal order from legal
analysis leading to targeted threats.

social organizations are shifting to a network form of management, via internet, IT and AI, it seems timely to shift this model to how humans relate to nature, and each other. Why do we not do so? We still concentrate on seeking more effective means of threating via tougher legal orders.

Much of this book was submitted to the Systems Sciences Program, Wharton School of Business, University of Pennsylvania as a dissertation. Back then, it was controversial. It is presented again to see if the controversy continues. Most university-based scientists saw it as speculation on the hopeless. They argued that there were economic measures to quickly correct the problem of deterioration, if indeed there was a problem. Some went deeper to point out that if the environment deteriorated to the extent projected, beyond economics, then society could shift to tougher and more threatening regulations via collective political will. Now, as the deterioration situation arrives, political leaders mostly go into hiding beneath it.

The 1979 work showed how more and tougher legislation would not solve problems of deterioration. They were systemic and not understood in analysis. Perhaps there is now hope for change as there is greater appreciation of the systemic over the analytic and more evidence of the urgency for change. Against this is the considerable evidence that the reasons for hopelessness are omnipresent. Many humans still portray nature as irrelevant to their life, or its enemy. The disrespect for nature and others is now more clearly seen as disrespect of self, within the dilemma of selfishness.

The research noted a shortcoming in managers relating to themselves. This stood in the way of genuine human concern for environmental deterioration. Changing the shortcoming in 1979 was thought outside the capability of regulation. In 2019 it seems beyond management, as well as scientific, technological, and industrial capabilities.

Mentioning concern for climate change from environmental deterioration in 1979 often halted a conversation. The Head of the US EPA sent me a letter in 1979 along with all copies of my reports that EPA had located in EPA saying? "We have no further use of these reports, your research, or you. I will ensure no government funding ever supports your further research."

Today, the subject often starts conversations but usually turns to much acrimony on all sides of the concern. Some, mostly scientists, fear there will be no human future on the planet. Others, mostly consultants to business, become angry at any call for radical changes to business as usual due to projected disasters. The second group quote from many sources, including the Bible, to argue why nature is a resource to be used at human will. Some argue how business as usual practices, with masculine leadership, are sacrosanct to human life. Others become very angry about any arguments of moving to business as unusual. They see it as a door to anarchy, with anarchy defined as a bad, as the French and Americans so define it. This differs from the rest of the world, including the Greeks that defined the idea. As such, concepts of how humans relate to each other, and themselves, seals the problem for how they relate to nature. Our hope in 2019 is that some of the world's leading businesspeople[81] are already operating well into the world of business as unusual.

---

[81] These would include the leaders of such firms as IKEA, China State Construction, and a few IT companies.

X

2019-DETERIORATION INTO CLIMATE CHANGE

1. 1979 – It's Too Early

In 1979, the dean of the Wharton School was upset with the project described herein. He did not see environmental deterioration as a concern for business. He thought students should concentrate on learning business as usual before going off and speculating on Hawk's "business as unusual." He was also concerned about examination of anarchy as self-regulation, which Hawk had called organizational self-governance of the "network form." Reviewers of the research noted that environmental deterioration did seem to be better managed via the expanded innovation encouraged by the network form of organization. That dean's appraisal was not his fault. His Wharton Advisory council was mostly American, and firmly tied to business as usual. They were protecting a legacy.

1979 business leadership in general was closely aligned with a Catholic tradition of management responsibility via tightly fixed hierarchies. For them, the emergence of Information Technology was thought to be something of temporary science fiction but in the long term may help them firm up the hierarchy of control. (They were right about the second.) The environmental deterioration research as done in factory operation management hierarchies was valuable in showing Maslow, and his model for improving management via a hierarchy, were wrong. Even the research and advice of Herbert Simon showing hierarchies were essential was seen to be wrong. In their management systems the workers would comment, "It's not my problem," and go home. Within the Eric Trist type autonomous workgroup, as seen the study, their likely response to a pollution problem was: "We need to fix this, any ideas?"

Many in the study expressed concern about the meaning of life beyond the fight of man versus nature. They asked if there were approaches to life that could avoid the war against nature they were involved in, and that resulting in environmental deterioration? Perhaps humans cannot manage such change? In attempting to bring humility to being human, Stephen Hawking points out:

> *"The human race is just a chemical scum on a moderate-sized planet, orbiting around a very average star in the outer suburb of one among a hundred billion galaxies. And that I can't believe the whole universe exists for our benefit. That would be like saying that you would disappear if I closed my eyes."* [82]

The dominant purpose herein is to redevelop the idea of regulation in a way that can enhance the opportunities for the desirable potentials of mankind to emerge, not threaten what is seen as undesirable. Current modes of social regulation predominantly attempt to restrict the undesirable characteristics of humans. Several modes of social regulation are outlined and investigated in this dissertation with respect to their ability to control complex societal problem issues.

The focus for the dissertation is environmental deterioration. The environment is conceptually analyzed in terms of man's relations to nature, the man-made environment, other men, and himself, (no disrespect is intended towards women as the term men is used as an abbreviation of mankind in general). This conceptual scheme

---

[82] Hawking, *Stephen*, *"Reality on the Rocks"* TV series (AP), aired, March 6, 2016.

is narrowed down with an empirical research focus on the specific domain of attempts to regulate pollution from industrial production facilities.

As there is a final research report available from the research project which this dissertation is based on, the empirical evidence is only outlined in this document. The research report is titled "Environmental Protection: Analytical Solutions in Search of Synthetic Problems," 1977. The report is available from the Institute of International Business at the Stockholm School of Economics, Stockholm, Sweden. The author is the same as of this dissertation.

The dissertation is the conceptual result of the research reporting. It had pointed to difficulties in the operation of environmental protection. The dissertation placed those difficulties within a context. Many of the difficulties relate to the extensive use of the mode of regulation I shall call Legalism, which is inappropriate for describing complexity. An alternative mode of regulation is formulated and proposed within the dissertation which offers a more desirable response to complexity. The alternative mode I have called Appreciation.

This document stands alone conceptually, with the empirical basis in the three volume original reports as done at the Institute of International Business, in Stockholm, Sweden. It chronicles economic motivations leading to industrialization practices that end in deterioration of the environment, the environment humans depend on. Each practice is seen to have strong economic argumentation, when see in bi-polar studies. Business as unusual would instead make use of the "both plus more" attitude and model of synthesis. In business-as-usual evidence is used to ensure facts showing how one side is right, usually the side that pays for the study. With business as unusual, the management function looks beyond the hoped-for results and includes the longer-term consequences as part of the price. The process begins in can it be true, then is it true for me, then what can we do about it? Humans seem unready to avoid the consequences of their actions resulting in deterioration.

Clearly, human activities on earth have led to deterioration of its environment in terms of loss of biodiversity, pollution, depletion of natural resources, massive landscape conversion to artificial uses, defaunation, and a warming climate.[83] Business as usual practices will soon lead to no business between humans and nature. What is most difficult to appreciate about all this is that as the consequences of some actions become clearer, we humans seem to expand them and emphasize doing the wrong things more efficiently, not exploring what innovation of the alternative can achieve. "It's Too Late," is used in a special way in this book. This point will be examined in more detail later, but somehow human hope springs from feeling a threat is so omnipresent as to define hopelessness in its too late. Once its perceived to be too late in a human setting leadership goes into hiding, or falls back, thus giving the opportunity to experiment with business as unusual.

Can someone instead prepare to write a different book, one that picks of the pieces of the past that are not linked to deterioration, and that allows for a tunnel of hope out of this mess and towards a new future? In theory it could all have been different, yet why was in not different? The "United Nations' Intergovernmental Science-Policy Platform on Biodiversity and Ecosystem" panel report concluded that about 10% of the 8.7 million living organisms will soon go extinct due to activities set up to serve humans.[84] From that scary beginning, the rate of demise is to expand.

We see several forces in serious conflict. Humans are at the center. We choose to fight with nature, each other, and ourselves. Perhaps resolution of these humanly inspired conflicts awaits the results of ongoing arguments with ourselves? us. The major conflict found herein is between the artificial of the industrial and the natural aspects of our environment. The conflict begins with minor deterioration, gains strength and breadth to disrupt and destroy systems of life, of which humans are connected. Humans, in general, feel something is wrong but can't see it because years of education and social training have brought them to filter out seeing the arrogance of humanistic. They can only see cause-effect relations in three dimensions but cannot conceive of the consequences playing out in the

[83] E. Stokstad, *Science* 364, p. 517-518, 2019.
[84] J. Tollefson, *Nature* 569, p. 171, 2019.

fourth dimension. They do see where it begins in one dimensional thinking of my point, or your point, but no connection, and ultimately settle on no point. All this is fixed in two dimensions to suit human laws and legally drawn legislation. This creates a fateful situation fixed in a natural time that naturally changes. Thus, it becomes troubled as it erratically catches up, i.e., changes, with troubles being more rapidly created.

Humans engineered the dilemma of life via industrialization being done in by the same. This is followed by lawyers attempting to fix it in two-dimensional actions from one-dimensional idea. Living systems need more than this. They need new ideas of the normative, repositioning humans as of and with nature. This can be a both plus more to move on to the more and allow it to manage the third dimension in terms of knowledge of the fourth. From this vision we must reorient the education of engineers, and then lawyers, to be consistent with a world of both plus more, not cause-effect inscribed in two dimensions based on one dimensional thinking that eventually becomes pointless.

Much hope for humans is now vested in Artificial Intelligence (AI) rising to compensate for the seeming lack of natural intelligence (NI). What was learned in the research behind this book is we perceive problems threatening our future then look for solutions that will solve the problems without disturbing the business as usual that supports our status quo. Technological solutions seem to offer "fixes" that seemingly do not change the context, i.e., insure changelessness.

As with conceptions of environmental protection, environmentalism, recycling, and sustainability, new human activities seem insignificantly innovative to allow an appreciation of nature. In the 1970's some of us defined an environmentalist as someone who bought their summer home last year. Recycling is mostly a tactic to retain trust in business as usual, industrial production and rabid growth in consumption. This begins in belief that the normal costs to the environment can be "recycled." This is a problem even if the environmental costs of collection and remanufacturing are ignored or given a discount for hearts in the right place. More questionable in the recycling process are the entropy cost built into the initial product designs and uses. Recycling mistakes does not eliminate the mistakes behind the mistakes. As scientists of the status of Einstein and Hawking long ago pointed out, the Second Law of Thermodynamics is sacrosanct in our universe. Soda cans are no more recyclable than humans are.

Two challenges have come to define the human future. These will become clarified as humans perceive a need to change how they define their conditions of life. The current perception is an artifact of 19th Century Newtonian-inspired industrialization, designed as a mechanical system that can eliminate or at least compensate for natures' irregularities. The industrial is managed with principles consistent with the industrial paradigm and its mechanization and operates in opposition to the vagaries of the larger environment. The results have been somewhat impressive. The longer-term consequences of these results seem to be great, perhaps greater than life can afford.

There is a growing need to rethink industry and its impact on the larger environment. The consequences of its operations are becoming significant. A rethink can begin in the seemingly trivial practices imbedded in human resource management, as taught in business schools, and practiced in their graduates. An example could be the Maslow 1943 Harvard business school human resource management theory for worker and societal motivation.[85] Beginning there can shine a new light on industrial processes and their role in deteriorating the relations between humans and the nature upon which they rely. Let us begin with a small look at this means of managing humans as resources for the industrial.

From research into humans as resources for industrialization, Maslow came up with a relatively perverse management form titled "hierarchy of human needs." It was to help managers motivate lower humans to move up through a hierarchy of accomplishments. Such was needed to induce natural beings to spend life in unnatural settings. Human resource management thus becomes party to a larger environmental deterioration problem, working in the service

---

[85] "A Theory of Human Motivation," *Psychology Review*, Abraham Maslow, Harvard, 1943.

to manipulating natural beings to function in industrialization settings. The environmental deterioration challenge is much wider than smoke from a coal-fired power plant. It involves much of what we define as civilization.

Going deeper into this seeming triviality, we see how Maslow's hierarchy becomes used to encourage humans to work ever-harder to access goods to meet their bio-physical needs. Then, the problem expands as humans strive to expanded possession of the results of industrial production. This process is organized towards the top of Maslow's hierarchy. Workers come to believe if they work harder, they will access increased power and/or wealth and become "self-actualized."[86] Herein lies the basis for humans expanding the problems of industrialization from meeting limited human needs to the grasping for human wants.

There were obvious problems with this model. Must strategic deceit be used to get natural beings to occupy unnatural settings for much of their lives? Why place an idea like self-actualization atop a hierarchy in that they rightfully are irrelevant to each other? Does this not further the problems in the ongoing war of humans against nature, via industrial? To date the accumulated wealth gained from progress up the hierarchy is seldom connected to self-actualization; it's mostly used to insulate those who can't find self-actualization and are bothered by it. As such, the idea of self-actualization has been translated to ideas about the mission of life being the acquisition of ever more "stuff;" as produced via industrialization. The result is an ever-expanding industrial basis to serve society's needs and wants.

The research outlined herein calls for a drastic rethink of industrialization, a mechanical process that is now at the core of the development and management of the human project and its consequential catastrophes. Posterity will be responsible for leading humans through the changing conditions of the two challenges. Some leader-

---

[86] There is much irony in this theory of organization. In it, hard work will propel you from grounded needs to ephemeral wants, and may allow access to the ultimate, self-actualization. In fact, those most referenced to have become self-actualized in the species were those who ignored or actively rejected fulfillment of ephemeral wants thereby finding higher priorities for life in nature.

ship participating in the research behind this work saw an ominous threat facing humans. They apparently were in a distinct minority.

The first challenge comes from many human activities being seen to *deteriorate* nature and the natural environment essential to a bio-systemic natural order. Central to this is the production and use of Petro-chemicals seen as essential to human activities even as they eliminate other species, and habitats. From the same homocentric attitude comes the destruction of air and water cleansing natural environments composed of trees, soils, oceans, lakes, ground waters and atmospheric conditions. Emerging knowledge warns humans of conditions of change via human activities at the earth's surface. These release CO_2 into the atmosphere thereby warming the atmosphere. The dire conditions created by this emerged from the work of a scientist in the study near its close in the fall of 1977, Dr. James F Black.

Most of the problems raised herein, and with humans in general, are relational. We must shift from vision based on and in analysis of parts, separated from context. We need a systems vision and approach to see relations, not parts pulled out and messed with, which create a larger mess when they are put back in their system; a system that had since moved on. Thus, relations and relationships are crucial to see, appreciate and manage. In this respect we look at relations between humans and nature, between humans and the built environments they surround themselves to protect the artificial from the natural, and between humans and other humans. All this stems from the most crucial of relations, the most difficult to repair and/ or manage: the relation to our self. The following diagram begins to outline the problem and the promise for change to business as unusual.

The challenge for humans is that their activities result in deterioration of the environmental conditions essential to their life and life on the planet. This poses a challenge to life as science defines it. As we learn more via science, we find less basis for optimism for continuation of that life which is presumed to be developed from science and technology.

Research shows a continual deterioration in the conditions of the natural environment due to human activities. Meanwhile, humans believe they are the crowning achievement of a cosmic trek called the human project. As such, humans continue to use, ignore, or degrade all species and systems of life; systems that are lesser in the hierarchy of life, as humans define it. This provides us with the ideology that we should *desecrate* nature, which becomes the logic for allowing and/or motivating deterioration of nature.

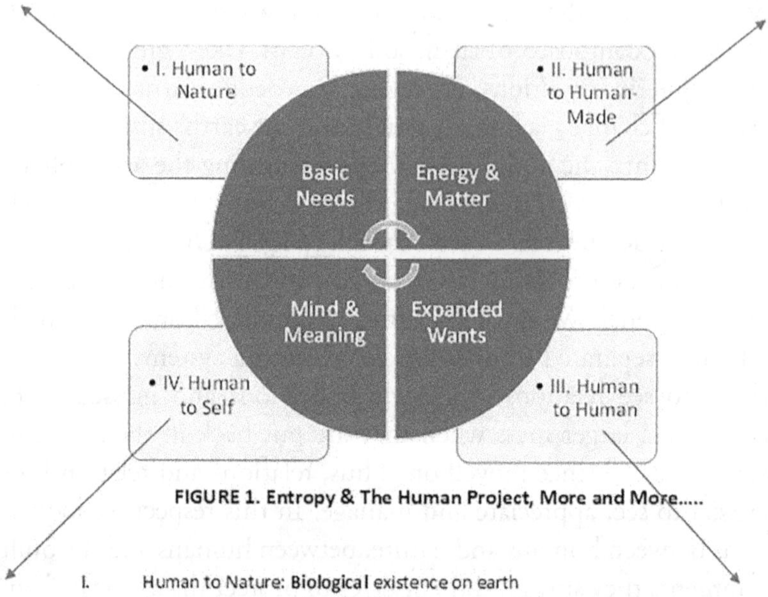

FIGURE 1. Entropy & The Human Project, More and More.....

I.   Human to Nature: **Biological** existence on earth
II.   Human to Human – Made: **Entropic** existence in the Cosmos
III.   Human to Human: **Social-political** activities
IV.   Human to Self: **Meaning of life** introspection (mentally fu_ked up)

Ideas in one domain profoundly affect the other domains. The systemic emphasizes context, the analytic obscures connectivity in context. Domain I is of the systemic while Domain II is derived from the analytic. Domain I provides the human context, Domain II provides the dilemma addressed by environmental protection efforts. The Economics of Doman II increases entropic speed.

Desecration is an idea of a religious tone that serves short-term humanistic needs, and then, unfortunate human wants. Humans believing there are technological solutions to all harmful consequences from their ill-considered actions in meeting their needs illustrates the importance of humanistic ideas. The unfortunate process is justified in combining Adam Smith economics with Darwinian conceptions of competitive advantage, both of which sponsor a particular dream of human evolution. This leads to the ideas behind business as usual between humans and the sponsorship of a kind of *industrialization* to supply that business and the distribution of its goods and services.

Behind industrialization, and its desecration of nature, stands a) religious scriptures, b) economic theories, and c) legalistic weaknesses. Values of what we call humanism define the value of all three while ensuring continuous deterioration of nature. These issues emerged from the research interviews as rationales for why change would be difficult, maybe impossible?

a) Justification for activities of humans that deteriorate are seen in religious texts. They emphasize the lowly role of nature relative to human aspirations: *"Be fruitful and multiply, and fill the earth, and subdue it; and rule over the fish of the sea and over the birds of the sky and over every living thing that moves on the earth."*[87] Most religions teach humans to aspire to and work under this belief.

b) Economic ideologies presume the value of an unfettered growth of production, distribution, and consumption. As worshippers of *The Economist* teachings firmly believe, increased productivity is the ultimate measure of a business enterprise, where deterioration consequences are expected, are usually insignificant, and can be managed via price, if ever needing to be managed. Few economists of the western tradition agree with Nicholas Georgescu-Roegen, that economic acts are entropy-aiding.

c) The role of legal process is seen as outside the pathways of ethics and truth, while forcefully directing humans to abide by laws with a questionable foundation. For example, the traditional legal process requires paper, very much paper. Thousands of trees are destroyed to

---

[87]   *The Bible*, Genesis, 1:26-30

provide two-dimensional platforms ordering obedience to one-dimensional ideas. Questions about the illogic of "humans protecting the environment from humans" are ignored within that dimension. There are problems with humans being human.

2. 2019 – It's Too Late

Stepping back, to see the environment more holistically and systemically, shows the danger of using segmented, analytic efforts to manage a larger, holistic phenomenon, such as the environment. It seems to add to its deterioration. Analyzing a systemic problem, to find its cause, generally expands it. We need to understand this, and appreciate the resulting dilemma, then find innovative ways out of it. As such, this is the second challenge herein. The difficulties become more complex as we find examples of effects preceding causes, as seen in early cybernetics. As such, nature can be more interesting than the science that attempts to know her.

Behind this second challenge, research reveals a deep human belief in future hope in what is being called the artificial. Defined via its abstraction from the natural it is lauded in books under the heading of "sciences of the artificial." Through it humans see a doorway to a better future, while its results to date are mostly seen to add to deterioration of the environment. The values behind the prominence of artificiality are due for a questioning. This will require an appreciation of what and how humans do what they do, especially under the flag of industrialization. In addition to the natural deterioration from nature's 2nd Law Entropic process[88] we add man-made processes of industrialization.

From this challenge to change we encounter a second challenge – it arises from serious concern for if, when and how humans can respond to the first challenge, that of deterioration of the natural

---

[88] Nicholas Georgescu-Roegen, "*The Entropy Law and Economic Progress,*" Harvard Press, 1971.

environment. Just now this is an economic discussion. Is there are way to effectively regulate the current definition of economic systems, or are there new ideas about the economics of nature?

Both challenges seem hard to visualize as dire and act up with speed. Interview data illustrated how urgency is masked by humanly creating complexities from false dichotomies. This leads to double binds and Catch 22s that form polarized debates about relations between man and nature, man and man, and man and self. One such debate stems from a dichotomy in a war between man and nature, where the two are in fact interdependent. This begins in the desecration of nature that leads to its deterioration. The internal war that sponsors the external war with nature is seen in immortality projects created to fight against the mortality intrinsic to the nature of life. Results of a study on which this is based show why and how societal approaches to regulation of individual human acts will not resolve either challenge; perhaps it is responsible for much that has come to be wrong between humans and their environments. With some urgency we need to move the human mentality towards authority via differences that make a beneficial difference.

The first challenge is to get humans to see that what they have done and are doing is a problem. The second challenge is how to deal with what was noticed, should it be noted before it's too late. The following illustrates the pervasiveness of the challenges in business as usual. It describes how a serious effort to rethink the costs of "business as usual" to the natural environment by human activities, was derailed in practices of real-time accounting for the sake of ever shorter-term profitability. Humans have long had a problem with their environment.

Many humans argue that they will always find ways to avoid a fateful conclusion, based on more extensive analysis, except of course for the systemic aspects of their own death, and/or enjoining a religious apocalypse, and, of course, the cosmic entropic conclusion. None-the-less, humans like to think of themselves as separate from nature, and even above nature. They find ways to ignore all evidence that they are linked to or even dependent upon nature. A group of humans argue that their actions cannot have unfortunate consequences. When evidence of the unfortunate meets their reality, they turn to investing recourses in order to obscure copiability. Why is it this way?

Via a business-as-usual attitude. change is defined in the manner that would suit the dwellers in the "Plato's Cave," as depicted in "The Allegory of the Cave." Families, schools, companies, governments, and other social institutions support the bias towards retention of business as usual at all costs. Just now the costs seem to be significantly growing.

Two hundred years of industrialization via science implies that humans can solve all problems, even those that result from technological solutions to non-technology problems. Regardless, the human project moves forward from a deep belief that humans will solve any and all problems. Thus, we arrive at the religion of humanism – a creed that humans have an ever-expanding power to control their reality while eliminating any and all challenges from it. Reexamination of humanism and its attitude towards the natural environment may be essential to finding beneficial change. Are humans capable of such self-reflection? Science shows us that change is a key definer of nature. Can humans ever accept change?

The social bonding forces of cultures and their traditions bind social organizations, but the price they pay is to consistently resist change. Attitudes want to be fixed and practices follow the values that structure attitudes. The common expression about this within a business is "Around here we do it this way. If you are uncomfortable with this perhaps you should look elsewhere." Diversity is seldom seen as an asset. As was often mentioned in the research interviews, as the reason for continuance of business as usual, "We do it this way because we always did it this way." Humanism helps to avoid seeing emerging problems to humans and their conditions of life. This was most clearly seen in the efforts of those trained in law schools in the US. Evidence of the end state of the written law can now be seen in the way the seemingly most intelligent lawyers compose their words to end as regulations. Contemporary environmental laws rely on ever longer paragraphs, sentences, and words.[89] It's as if these individuals' sense that the system they are educated to work in is now working thus they mask the problem by using 125 plus word sentences. It's as if they don't know how to begin a statement and wish to avoid ending it.

Humanists counter change by arguing how change is always taking place, thus it is a constant, thus it can be ignored. In this way change is strangely defined as permanence. Relative to climate change the humanist ideology mistakenly argues that weather (which is not climate change) is always changing, thus it's a constant and climate change doesn't matter. For them, what then is the problem? From interviews in the study behind this work it seemed that the more ominous a change facing humans, the more openly they would ignore it. Their creed was that it's best to simply ignore change, as it will change away anyway and thus be gone. Except for the subject matter at hand, this seemed funny.

3. 2023: Now What?

-   After forty years the effects, then the causes of environmental deterioration, are being seen in science turned upside down, inside out, as it examines its history in building the industrialized environment of the artificial against the natural, that provided the world with the consequences known as deterioration of the natural.
-   Who will win in the war with nature? No one and nothing. Winning is a human construct. Entropy continues despite who and what humans are. Are humans a small problem restricted to planet earth? Can humans be anything more than a problem?

---

[89] This will be discussed later but it was common to see laws of hundreds of pages and sentences of 125 plus words where the authors seem to not know how to enter and why to exit a sentence. Many participants in the research on which this is based saw this as a lawyer joke in the reverse sense; where the joke was on those relying on the legal system to solve systemic problems.

- Where will humans go? Most likely, they will continue into the deeper and darker with much that is artificial to light the way into the unhappy darkness. It is as if humans are returning from where they escaped, back into Plato's Allegory of the Cave. Why do many humans prefer the changelessness advised by Parmenides and Confucius, and Plato, and avoid the ideas about a better chance in the change of Socrates and Lao Tzu, and then Heraclitus? Why do most humans not know of those who set the stage for unaided rationality, industrialization, then deterioration?
- Cultural institutions and social organizations must shift to explicit questioning of business as usual in a human search for beneficially innovative business as unusual. Schools with their youth very interested in a future public good can be leaders in this. Most teachers are ready for such, if they could set the rules that encourages the innovative to replace the tried and truly wrong.
- Learn to be nice to each other and nature, we are all in this together.
- Redesign your life and the infrastructure that connects. Fewer airplane trips, more public transit, especially high-speed rail to connect the part of the earth. A conference was held in 1991 on this; "Conditions of Success: Grand Hotel, Stockholm."
- Good night and Good luck.

The history of human relations to nature is interesting. Humans were and are biologically linked to nature. They depend on the well-being of an environment they share with nature for conditions of life. While some humans seem aware of this, many ignore or openly reject it during their lives. The evidence for this is seen everywhere in their choices about life and manner of living. As such, there should be a deep concern for the human future. There is not. A recent attempt to modify the human attitude towards nature came in environmental protection regulation. Sadly, the mostly legal then governance activities have signified a continuation of the traditional attitude towards nature. A few problems were resolved but those could have been addressed in more efficient and effective ways. The topic herein moves beyond ideas of the natural environment needing human protection. Interest herein is centered on the longer-term consequences of nature's relations back to humans, more than humans arrogantly attempting to protect nature from human activities planned to continue.

Man's history is written in terms of relations to nature although more concentrates on human-to-human history. That which involved nature seldom mentioned humans causing environment deterioration. This changed with humanly directed scientific discovery, especially our accessing the science of erasing humans via nuclear war, or development of chemicals dangerous to life. Thirty years later, we see danger signs from more widespread problems in the long-term consequences of industrialized pollution becoming near-term hazards to life. Just now there is new research posing that the consequences could end up changing planetary conditions, the conditions essential to life. Just now this is introduced as "climate change." Thus, the relations to nature are growing much more serious than mutual creation of life or the accommodating the hostility to nature in her irreversible processes of entropic death.

To organize their opposition to nature humans developed what we will call the "human project." Its mission was and is to gain control over natural processes then nature or replace her with the artificial. Underlying this project humans wish to find meaning in the limits of human life. One means is to work to create neg-entropy in defiance of natural entropy. Via their passion for this project humans work to develop ways to avoid, ignore, denounce and/or destroy what nurtures them.

Why do humans praise artificial things and de-link themselves from nature and the natural systems of life? It seems rejecting nature is essential to growing up, much like teenagers rejecting their home and family to go off and development meaning of self, via selfishness. Such human logic has long been responded to in religious dogmas and business school texts. Is it assumed to be important to human development to do such? Perhaps it's only a distraction to avoid seeing ethical shortcomings of humans involved in conflict and destruction? Or it's a way to put entropic death outside a passion for life.

Clearly, many humans have a negative attitude towards nature. This attitude begins in the religion of environmental desecration and moves into environmental deterioration. Perhaps it is a self-imposed suicide of the species via explicit destruction of its essential context? Clearly there is some form of self-destructive process underway as evidenced by environmental deterioration from human activities. The process has grown from background noise to a noticeable and then noteworthy threat. How much further must it expand before it can mobilize humans to upgrade the mythology of human purpose and its artificial meanings?

Just now, in 1979, we seem to be approaching a crucial moment in history. We face some fateful choices about life and human activities to support or deny that life on the planet. There are early signs of a need to create a new myth around which to organize the human project. Hope lies mostly with the young. The work presented herein is mostly for them, as they will carry the cost of the elder's errors in judgement and practices.

XI

RELATIONS BETWEEN NATURE
AND HUMAN NATURE

The following is about a war. We need to gain a clearer sense of who or what we humans are, and what we strive to become, or at least do. We want to win but are not sure against who or what. We often are at work against other humans but underlying this we seem at war against nature, including nature in ourselves. In so doing we praise the artificial.

Humans have negotiated with nature for most of their existence. Intimate collaborations over creation of life, hostility about the march to death, and general misunderstands of what nature is have sustained an interesting one-sided discourse. Humans arise from nature while remaining biologically dependent on her and of course her well-being until their death. Humans act with much arrogance and little appreciation for nature, and what she represents in the universe.

In this, it seems appreciation is key to beneficial change. As used here, appreciative systems come from the social sciences work by Sir Geoffrey Vickers. He outlined the importance of this missing attitude in his 1965 "The Art of Judgement" book. He then elaborated in more detail on why we need to learn appreciation in his 1970 book: "Freedom in a Rocking Boat: Changing Values in an Unstable Society." Appreciation, as Vickers presented it, was key to his framework for how to change what we value, then now to upgrade values via a wider appreciation of context. He argued how we make decisions from values while modifying the decisions while leaving the values driving them unquestioned.

Systemic appreciation can lead towards self-management. It can point to the need for self-limiting, self-reversing and openness to redefinition. This opens the door to upgrading via allowing for fluid and open processes. Vickers's appreciative systems seem ideal to encourage human nature to come to appreciate the nature of nature.

> "Learning what to want is the most radical, the most painful and the most creative art of life." (Freedom in a Rocking Boat, 1970, from the introduction). [90]

This underlines the need to transform the process of humans working to meet their needs then coming to expand that work into processes of expanding into seemingly unrestricted wants. This is primarily done via discovery and development of industrialization and the areas of science set up to feed it. This has allowed a shift from direct human experience with nature to building and expanding on the world of the artificial. This encourages humans in failing to appreciate nature and initiate activities such as leveling parts of a forest to build a housing development that removes much nature and then brings deterioration to the remaining nature. To obscure this process, humans invent mythologies around the importance of "human projects." These projects, such as an expansive one called industrialization, seeks meaning for humans by transforming the "is of the natural" into the "human idea of what ought to be." The current stage of this human project has been called "post-industrialization." It is clearly even more industrial than post but more significant herein is how it lacks appreciation of nature at an even more expansive level. It illustrates a muddled dichotomy in human thinking. It espouses actions to protect the natural environment from human

---

[90] Vickers, Geoffrey, Freedom in a Rocking Boat, Penguin Books: Middlesex, England, 1970.

actions but therein introduced a self-reinforcing contradiction in values with no obvious escape.

This industrialization human project has introduced a more extensive de-appreciation of any former signs of appreciation of nature. It did this via an enthusiastic denouncing, ignoring, avoiding and/or destruction of nature. It's an unhappy situation for systems nurtured by nature. The question then becomes why do humans want to de-link themselves from nature and the systems of life that define nature? Is moving out from nature a good thing, like teenage humans moving out from home, parents, and background. In many religious dogmas and business school texts there is an image of nature as an economic resource that should be used in support of human ends.

Why is our attitude towards nature so uncaring or negative? Our attitude goes from environment as something to overpower, to something to desecrate. In both activities we work to deteriorate nature via our relations with it. Thus, we carry out destruction of the context of life. While being part of life we thus carry out a self-destructive process. While acting to increase environmental deterioration via our activities we endanger ourselves. The consequences are now noticeable. Soon they will become devastating.

Is it possible for humans to create a new mythology from a new human purpose? Can we come to appreciate nature as fundamental to life? We are just now approaching the moment in human history when such choices matter. There are signs of recognizing a need for a new myth to guide human development. The following work is mostly for the youth, as they will carry the cost of the elder's manifest errors in judgement and practice.

Herein I disregard the excuse of human's incompetence and thus their need for forgiveness. The human attitude towards nature and the supporting actions are clearly derogatory and now sufficiently dangerous to the context of life to require urgent change. What can be done, how should humans change, where should change begin? Let's begin with the dominant problem solver of modern society, regulation. This has become the general means to respond to evidence of a societal wrong being done. From bi-polar beliefs and/or analytically filtered evidence regulation is drawn up by those with limited beliefs, no science and analytic filtration as acquired in law schools. This is done in the cause of creating social regulation against the cause of the effect. Western society is quite proud of the results of this for organizing and improving society. It has been attempted for about a decade in use to slow and then reverse environmental deterioration processes. The evidence for what this brought society comes from the research project mentioned above.

Regulation efforts are seen in the factories, refineries and company headquarters that assisted with the research behind this writing. The evidence shows regulation to have missed the contextual issues, usually done very late, and often turned counterproductive. My responses come from evidence in a two-year research study of various national systems of regulating environmental protection. Some who helped with the study believe it may now be too late although it may appear too early. These included those in industry who knew most about the role of industrial by-products and how they don't, as in the minds of some legally educated politicians in the United States, simply disappear if a law is passed to dispense with their potential for harm to life. In addition, there were government officials with calm insight into the pending problem for living systems in continuation of business as usual and believed we cannot long afford factions arguing over how much pollution is tolerable. One member from industry, an American, argued that current industrial practices will lead to fundamental change in our planet's climate. Two regulators, one each from Canada and Sweden, went deeper to argue that we in essence are dependent on a support system that will soon encounter planetary deterioration at an unresolvable scale. At that point solutions like pollution catchment, limits on population growth, halting destruction of natural terrain will seem small to irrelevant. No regulators trained in the law ever voiced such a concern in the project.

Humans have come to occupy a parallel world that they have created mostly from and in two dimensions. It is commonly known as the world of the artificial. In it we occupy an artificially constructed habitat that we define as superior to living in nature. We often go so far as believing the artificial is superior to living "with" nature. Where does this human want arise from? Is it genetic or acquired via mental constructs? Why do humans feel they want to or even need to be distant from nature?

Perhaps the ideology arises from the mentality of myths. If so, this will be difficult to address in that myths are often the unquestioned untruths of societies. Humans deeply feel they need to oversee their place in the world, a feeling that easily becomes a passion for overseeing the world as they know it. We have developed a mythology that somehow guides us into opposition of nature. This is ironic, or tragic, in that we also know life is defined by and dependent upon nature. Perhaps since nature defined life to end in death, we do not trust nature, thus we are born in conflict with her? If true, this insight may give access to the world of human dilemmas in the human condition. It thus presents humans with *the dilemma* of their life and may well be beyond their reconciliation. Perhaps this is the source of human religions as comforting mythologies, as well as rationalization of why throwing a plastic bottle and cheeseburger wrapper out the window is a sign of strength, not simply being filthy.

Dilemmas are like Joseph Heller's *Catch-22*, where you are damned if you do or you don't, no matter what. It is also like Gregory Bateson's *double-bind that* invites schizophrenia in those caught up in it, especially if they are restricted to use of unaided-rationality. Or like West Churchman's depiction of the enemies of systemic thinking relying on that which is defined as rational, about 10% of Churchman's reality, while discounting or completely ignoring the other 90% in. This is ultimately what those concerned with the environment and our war with its natural governance face. Perhaps there is no way out. Elsewhere I've argued that we can start to resolve this via thinking in *both plus more* terms, where the rational and non-rational are combined to stand on in search of the vastly more insightful *more*. Herein I suggest we may find such in the 5th dimension that humans seem to have no access to.

Myth is here used in the sense of Joseph Campbell. He often lectured how myths are at the center of social-organizational thinking, be it for good or bad purposes. More succinctly, he suggested *myths are public dreams, while dreams are private myths*. Myths organize the elements that define the human condition and then the actions and activities that bring it about. Leading myths become societal stories that lead to satisfying human needs with echoes that expand to deal with human wants. Currently mythology is clearly connected to dreams of an industrial state organized by the sciences of the artificial. As we see how the current sense of industrialization is dangerous to the human context, we may well try to create a new myth. In the current situation we are entering a major dilemma with two aspects to it.

1. Relations to Nature

Part I is that nature is clearly not dependent on human wellbeing. Part II is that aspects of being human link back to present danger to nature's wellbeing, perhaps her survival. Arising from religious and cultural myths are stories and mentoring systems that favor ignoring nature or moving on to emphasize the un-natural dimension of life, the artificial. Within these myths are powerful entities that are not normally understandable except via the interpretations of a few humans, generally of the male version, that represent interpretations of nature via such myths as the Garden of Eden to explain nature.

Other humans, also men, offer an opposition myth that allows any to interpret the natural surroundings in a more objective manner, although any wishing to do so must accept the mythology of technology as generated via rational knowledge gained from science. Not that different from a religion, this approach leaves us with unaided rationality to deal with that which is not required to be rational. Humans thus lack appreciation for the non-rationality of nature from the choices of the chromosome to the essential need of black holes to allow the cosmos to make sense, even if it is sense beyond rationality. These myths pose problems for humans relating to nature and ever appreciating how their activities deteriorate the environment on which both depend.

"It was not until the working out of modern psychanalysis that we could understand something the poets and religious geniuses have long known; that the armor of character was so vital to us that to shed it meant to risk death and madness. It is not hard to reason out; If character is a neurotic defense against despair and you shed that defense, you admit the full flood of despair, the full realization of the true human condition, what men are really afraid of, what they struggle against, and are driven toward and away from."[91]

"As humans, we exist within a thin fabric of natural and artificial systems of order. During an earlier period of history man relied on non-scientific methods of relating to the natural order. Even though man felt that he could not then directly control natural processes, he felt he could indirectly participate in them by gaining favor with the "gods" in charge of nature (e.g., Sun "Rain God," etc.) The offering of sacrifice was one dominant made of "regulating" nature. Social orders were built around this mode of regulation, with prominence given to those men with the greatest potentials for communicating with the "gods, e.g., priests.

Through the efforts of men like Kepler, Copernicus, and Galileo, it was demonstrated that some natural processes could be explained with scientifically reasoned knowledge. Man's perception of communication with nature was moving into the realm of tangible, direct control. The age of discovering that mankind's reduction of uncertainties in our direct relations with nature might be responsible for increasing uncertainties in nature's indirect relations back to man. The environmental pollution aspects of the 1960s was one indication of the impact of the uncertainties. "[92]

---

[91] (Ernest Becker, *The Denial of Death*, New York: The Free Press, 1973, pp. 56-57)

[92] IBID

"Current discussion in very small circles about the twenty first century problems, called climate change as described in the work of Eunice Newton Foote in 1856, may illustrate a justifiable fear of what humans do that they fail to correct."[93]

The human attitude to nature might best be envisioned as derived from a religion of "homocentricity," sometimes called a "religion of humanism." This religion and its closely held beliefs may well be the definition of the problem of 1978.

"There is more than an academic reason for writing about the religious nature of humanism, for some of humanism's religious assumptions are among the most destructive ideas in common currency, a main source of the peril in this most perilous of epochs since the expulsion from Eden. Nor is the danger merely a potential one – to be characterized as the figment of a doomsday neurosis, and then dismissed.[94] Ehrenfeld then goes deeper. He seeks the underlying characteristics of humanism as seen in the dominant human myth.

Because human intelligence is the key to human success, the main task of the humanists is to assess its power and protect its prerogatives wherever they are questioned or challenged. Among the correlates of humanism is the belief that humankind should live for itself because we have the power to do so, the capacity to enjoy such a life, and nothing else to live for. Another correlation is the faith in the children of pure reason, science, and technology. Although shaken in recent years and the source of much confusion among humanists, this faith continues to permeate our existence.[1] and influence our behavior...[95]

[93] (David Hawk, *Regulation of Environmental Deterioration*, Philadelphia Pa, The Wharton School, U of Penn: S[3] Papers: #79-12, pp 24-25.)

[94] *The Arrogance of Humanism*, Ehrenfeld, David, New York: Oxford University Press, 1978, p. 4

[95] (Ibid., p. 5-6)

Relating Relationships

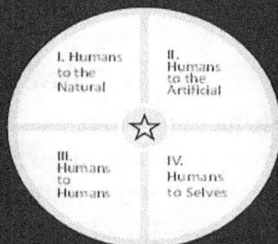

I. Humans to the Natural	II. Humans to the Artificial
III. Humans to Humans	IV. Humans to Selves

-Humans have difficulties in relating to nature, yet they also have difficulties in relations to the man-made, and with each other. Perhaps most serious is relating to self.

-Question: which domain offers a key access to understanding humans and deterioration?

Human Relations Quadrants

These are seen with great clarity in the work of Joseph Campbell in his inventory of human behavior that points towards the human passion to rise above nature and move towards an emphasis on tyranny, as it arises from the will to leadership in a society via the peculiarities of its culture.

> "The tyrant is proud, and therein resides his doom. He is proud because he thinks of his strength as his own; thus, he is in the clown role, as a mistaker of shadow for substance; it is his destiny to be tricked. ... The hero of yesterday becomes the tyrant of tomorrow unless he crucifies himself today."[96]

2. Deteriorating Nature To Create The Artificial

During thousands of years designing and developing what may be called the human project there has been a consistent desire to develop support systems to satisfy humans' needs. Although it was always a bit homocentric, humans recently emphasized the homocentric. In so doing they created a paradox where the current support

---

[96] Joseph Campbell, The Hero with a Thousand Faces, 1949, P. 289.

system for human life has become a major threat to all life. This change is outlined in the following. On the satisfying of insatiable human wants. Problems of managing consequences of meeting insatiable wants.

A) *The emergence of insatiable wants?* Humans have long enjoyed inventing and organizing machines to meet basic human needs. This has become widely known and accepted. This has come to be called industrialization. Based on its early success, the model expanded to attempt the satisfaction of essentially insatiable human wants. The collective results from this provide the consequences that increasingly challenge humans. All industrialization has some deterioration associated with it. Massive industrialization has massive consequences for its environment, and the conditions of life. Meeting human wants is not like the meeting of "more basic" bio-physical needs of life. Human wants are ill-defined and infinitely expansive. The watchword is "more." Many businesses are based on expanding this more.

Industrialization applies machine logic and mechanization to the provision of goods and services. In the beginning these are to meet tangible human needs.[97] Much of the labor required to maintain bio-life has been replaced with machines.

Industrialization responded to a call for more plentiful sources of food, water, and shelter, and served to allow expansion of the human population. This called for and allowed an exponentially expanding industrialization. This expansion was then squared with industrialization moving

---

[97] Now known as *cybernetics*, industrialization was also in the psyche of humans in Roman and prior eras of civilization creating. Coined by Norbert Wiener in 1948 as "theory or study of communication and control."

to also meet human wants. Wants are very different from the limitations found in the world of bio-physical needs. They are much more ambiguous, thus more ambitious. Our wants lack tangible limits and controls. In essence they are virtual[98] and easily move beyond methods of self-control. They can expand infinitely. Self-regulation, via the thinking of Socrates and Lao Tzu, offers the best form of managing human wants. Social regulation can be effective in managing bio-physical needs. Socrates talked of this distinction, as did Lao Tzu.

Serious dangers have accompanied the expanding ideas of the industrial and the artificial. Approaching consequences seem deep and dangerous. Dreams of reason have helped spur this development. We see serious threats to systems of life as they evolve on our planet. The systems depend on conditions for life, conditions that have long been deteriorating, but now approach a point of change beyond the capabilities of human management. The evidence for this in the study was strong. If true, then business as usual will come to represent no business. Even human needs will no longer be met.

B) *Problems of managing consequences of meeting insatiable wants.* If the first challenge, that industrialization emphasizes the problems between humans and nature, proves to be correct, then the second challenge is how humans deal with the changing conditions of life from challenge one. Industrialized changes can be clearly seen as detrimental to continuance of life. How then can or should humans respond to the situation prior to mortality? We know life is mortal, but does it need to be such at a more systemic level, say of a species? In addition, we know of the entropic

---

[98] Virtual is here used in the sense given it by Susanne Langer in *Form and Feeling*, 1953.

quality of all the universe and its contents. Entropy was not the concern of the research, although entropic processes emerged as important to the deterioration process being studied. Via entropy there is an essential deterioration underway regardless of human actions, presence, or absence. The problem, as confronted in this work, is that human actions, especially those associated with economic thinking for fulfilling human wants, seem only to add to the entropic process.[99] Per Georgescu-Roegen's work we see how virtually all economic thoughts and acts only speed the entropic process. So much so that human youth begin to see the industrial process as an entropy machine. If all this is so, then how can we hope to govern, regulate, control, or even deal with the first challenge as outlined above? This presents us with a second challenge. It is sufficiently serious as to take us beyond human capability to correct the industrial process. If we simply stop industrialization, a process at the center of our definition of the "good life," do we also stop that life?

Thinking in dimensional terms seemed helpful to explaining the results to some participants in the research. This was where charts were used to demonstrate how humans seem limited to thinking in one dimension at any time, as depicted by a line with two ends. This seems to have been a limitation through human history as seen in the limits of dichotomies, oppositions, politics, arguments, Catch-22s, ultimatums, etc. Humans tend to formalize conclusions from 0-dimensional thinking via 1-dimensional presentations, where with minimal thoughts a person stands at one end or the other of a line. The logic of the 0-dimension thus comes to be written as sacraments upon 2-D sheets of paper via those trained in the writing of legal documents, currently depicted as legalese, all after deciding on which end of the line to stand on, or for. Next, we act out our understand-

---

[99] The Entropy Law and The Economic Process, Nicholas Georgescu-Rogen, Harvard Press: Cambridge, 1971.

ing in a three-dimensional reality. The espoused end is enhancement of human life, and, less poetically, adding to the universal entropic process that manages all things as it moves them irreversibly in time into a 4th dimension. This implies that human's best hope appears to be moving regulation from the 2nd dimension into the 5th dimension, where humans cannot go.

If you can understand the above, you are smarter than I am. Regardless of my limits it is obvious that the challenges arise from systemic problems in connections, not those in parts as amenable to reductionistic analysis. Unfortunately, our education is in avoiding or not noticing that which is systemically connected. We continue to rely on industrialized analysis. This continues in the late 1940's development of cybernetic systems that now call for development of AI. The research shows there is no "post-industrial" transition underway. The research also shows this to be an important part of the environmental deterioration problem. The second challenge, how to manage the consequences of gaining intended and unthoughtful results, is large. Can the problem be managed by those who created it via their using the same analytic logic that created it?

Most humans seem to think yes, and support responses being called environmental protection regulation. We can regulate by making its existence illegal, as was done in New Jersey, or, more realistically, pose large threats upon those that create pollution if they do not manage it to make it harmless. We now begin to see from the study that the second, more realistic, option is also not part of any world we inhabit. Regulation begins with funding expensive and extensive research using the best analytic minds available to apply the best analytic models. A model of science is expected to arrive at the best methods of regulating. These have been shown to be effective as they analytically determine pre-determined causes of post-determined effects, all while applying the best of scientific methods from the 19th Century. Problems in this are now emerging.

If the problem is by its nature systemic then by definition it is set up to fail if guided by results of analytic thinking. Study results herein show that not only may it not manage the problem but may well worsen the situation of which the problem is only a part. Another approach is needed. Important herein are questions about values and value systems that lie underneath all of the above-mentioned choices.

Herein I disregard the excuse that humans are incompetent and in need of forgiveness. The human attitude towards nature and the supporting actions are clearly derogatory and now sufficiently dangerous in the context of life to require urgent change. What can be done, how should humans change, where should change begin? Let's begin with the dominant problem solver of modern society, regulation. This has become the general means to respond to evidence of a societal wrong being done. From bi-polar beliefs and/or analytically filtered evidence regulation is drawn up by those with limited beliefs, no science and analytic filtration as acquired in law schools. This is done in the cause of creating social regulation against the cause of the effect. Western society is quite proud of the results of this for organizing and improving society. It has been attempted for about a decade in use to slow and then reverse environmental deterioration processes. The evidence for what this brought society comes from the research project mentioned above.

Regulation efforts are seen in the factories, refineries and company headquarters that assisted with the research behind this writing. The evidence shows regulation was too little, done too late, and often seen as counterproductive? My responses come from evidence in a two-year research study of various national systems of regulating environmental protection. Some who helped with the study believe it may now be too late although to others it may appear too early. Those most concerned were industry representatives who knew most about the role of industrial by-products and how they don't just go away. On the other hand, the lawyers as politicians in the United States, simply disappeared once a law was passed, or commented in the study: "Sure, the law has problems, but we will put it out there for a year or two then bring it back in for repair. It's hard to predict these things." There were agency people that knew more and better. They would point to serious problems for living systems from laws as written from analysis that had been limited. They would comment on the continuous need they encountered in lowering what was the tolerable level of pollution and deterioration.

One member from industry, an American, argued that current industrial practices will lead to fundamental change in our planet's climate. Two regulators, one each from Canada and Sweden, went deeper to argue that we will soon encounter planetary deterioration at an unacceptable level, as well as unresolvable scale. At that point solutions like pollution catchment, limits on population growth, halting destruction of natural terrain, etc. will be irrelevant. It was interesting that in the study no regulators trained in the law ever voiced such a deep concern for the prospects of environmental deterioration.

Humans have come to occupy a parallel world that they have created mostly from and in two dimensions. It is commonly known as the world of the artificial. In it we occupy an artificially constructed habitat that we define as superior to living in nature. We often go so far as believing the artificial is superior to living "with" nature. Where does this human want arise? Is it genetic or acquired via mental constructs? Why do humans feel they want to or even need to be distant from nature?

Perhaps the ideology arises from the mentality of myths. If so, this will be difficult to address in that myths are often the unquestioned untruths of societies. Humans deeply feel they need to oversee their place in the world, a feeling that easily becomes a passion for overseeing the world as they know it. We have developed a mythology that somehow guides us into opposition of nature. This is ironic, or tragic, in that we also know life is defined by and dependent upon nature. Perhaps since nature defined life to end in death, we do not trust nature, thus we are born in conflict with her? If true, this insight may give access to the world of human dilemmas in the human condition. It thus presents humans with *the dilemma* of their lives and may well be beyond their reconciliation. Perhaps this is the source of human religions as comforting mythologies, as well as rationalization of why throwing a plastic bottle and cheeseburger wrapper out the window is a sign of strength, not simply being filthy.

Dilemmas are like Joseph Heller's *Catch-22*, where you are damned if you do or you don't, no matter what. It is also like Gregory Bateson's *double-bind that* invites schizophrenia in those caught up in it, especially if they are restricted to use of unaided-rationality. Or like West Churchman's depiction of the enemies of systemic thinking relying on that which is defined as rational, about 10% of Churchman's reality, while discounting or completely ignoring the other 90% in. This is ultimately what those concerned with the environment and our war with its natural governance face. Perhaps there is no way out. Elsewhere I've argued that we can start to resolve this via thinking in *both plus more* terms, where the rational and non-rational are combined to stand on in search of the vastly more insightful *more*. Herein I suggest we may find such in the 5th dimension, where humans are excluded.

Myth is here used in the sense of Joseph Campbell. He often lectured how myths are at the center of social-organizational thinking, be it for good or bad purposes. More succinctly, he suggested *myths are public dreams, while dreams are private myths*. Myths organize the elements that define the human condition and then the actions and activities that bring it about. Leading myths become societal stories that lead to satisfying human needs with echoes that expand to deal with human wants. Currently mythology is clearly connected to dreams of an industrial state organized by the sciences of the artificial. As we see how the current sense of industrialization is dangerous to the human context, we may well try to create a new myth. In the current situation we are entering a major dilemma with two aspects to it.

Part I is that nature is clearly not dependent on human wellbeing. Part II is that aspects of being human link back to present danger to nature's wellbeing, perhaps her survival. Arising from religious and cultural myths are stories and mentoring systems that favor ignoring nature or moving on to emphasize the un-natural dimension of life, the artificial. Within these myths are powerful entities that are not normally understandable except via the interpretations of a few humans, generally of the male version, that represent interpretations of nature via such myths as the Garden of Eden to explain nature.

Other humans, also men, offer an opposition myth that allows any to interpret the natural surroundings in a more objective manner, although any wishing to do so must accept the mythology of technology as generated via rational knowledge gained from science. This has become something of a religion thus it leaves us with unaided rationality to deal with that which is not required to be rational. Humans thus lack appreciation for the non-rationality of nature from the choices of the chromosome to the essential need of black holes to allow the cosmos to make sense, even if it is sense beyond rationality. These myths pose problems for humans relating to nature and ever appreciating how their activities deteriorate the environment on which both depend.

The human attitude to nature might best be envisioned as derived from a religion of "homocentricity," sometimes called a "religion of humanism." This religion and its closely held beliefs may well be the definition of the problem of 1978.

> "There is more than an academic reason for writing about the religious nature of humanism, for some of humanism's religious assumptions are among the most destructive ideas in common currency, a main source of the peril in this most perilous of epochs since the expulsion from Eden. Nor is the danger merely a potential one – to be characterized as the figment of a doomsday neurosis, and then dismissed.[100]

Ehrenfeld then goes deeper. He seeks the underlying characteristics of humanism as seen in the dominant human myth.

> Because human intelligence is the key to human success, the main task of the humanists is to assess its power and protect its prerogatives wherever they are questioned or challenged. Among the correlates of humanism is the belief that humankind should live for itself because we have the power to do so, the capacity to enjoy such a life, and nothing else to live for. Another correlation is the faith in the children of pure reason, science, and technology. Although

---

[100] Ehrenfeld, David, *The Arrogance of Humanism*, New York: Oxford University Press, 1978, p. 4

shaken in recent years and the source of much confusion among humanists, this faith continues to permeate our existence and influence our behavior....[101]

These are seen with great clarity in the work of Joseph Campbell in his inventory of human behavior that points towards the human passion to rise above nature and move towards an emphasis on tyranny, as it arises from the will to leadership in a society via the peculiarities of its culture.

"The tyrant is proud, and therein resides his doom. He is proud because he thinks of his strength as his own; thus he is in the clown role, as a mistaker of shadow for substance; it is his destiny to be tricked."– (Joseph Campbell, The Hero with a Thousand Faces, P. 289).....“The hero of yesterday becomes the tyrant of tomorrow, unless he crucifies himself today." [102](Ibid, p. 303)

3. Meaning of The Artificial

Nature furnishes the external environment. Humans use parts of this environment to gather resources to create their own more private, homocentric environment. This is an artificial environment, one that humans appear to be proud of. Additionally, nature provides humans with their internal and evolving genetic code. From this breadth of relations why then would humans hold nature in such disrespect. Where would we look for answers to this great dilemma? To address this, we need to look more seriously at the innovative breakthroughs that brought so many benefits and so much power to improving the human condition. This begins with the thinking of an Englishman, Sir Isaac Newton, and his impact on designing an industrial revolution. This brought artificially construed, rational

---

[101] (Ibid., p. 5-6)
[102] (Ibid, p. 303)

processes to humans meeting human needs. The process centered on a need to provide for bio-needs but rapidly expanded to meeting large needs associated with human life on earth, i.e., shifting from meeting needs to allow expansion of wants. This addresses long standing concerns for finding meaning in life. This allowed a means to answer questions such as: why we are here, where do we come, where to do we go, what matters, etc.

There is clearly a mismatch between natural processes and human activities. In the early 1960s the mismatch became more apparent and was labeled as environmental deterioration. The human response to continuing deterioration was environmental protection regulations. Once regulated, humans continued adding to the initial problem via homocentric economics, seeming to not realize that deterioration and economics were interconnected. Natural resources continued as widely available and freely accessible inputs to an economic mechanism set up to meet human needs then provide for human wants. Most human lives were and still are employed in the entertainment of seeking and meeting wants beyond needs. An economic myth directs and manages the process, where myth is herein used in the non-derogative manner of Joseph Campbell. Via their myth of economic process humans work hard to formulate and attain economic ends. Unfortunately, there are problems in this myth. They used to show up as deterioration. Now they are becoming more serious.

There are serious limitations in the economic and scientific logic of two hundred years ago. This guides the way humans take resources from nature to use as inputs to economic realizations. The cost to nature for providing inputs necessary to what we call the economic process was discounted greatly, then simply disregarded. This began in an attitude towards nature written by men in early biblical teachings and then became firmed up in the later ideologies of Adam Smith and Isaac Newton. In this, there was a fundamental mismatch in human perception and natural reality. The major costs for the mismatch may well be about to come due. Can humans respond effectively, then survive the costs? Now the mismatch between nature and humans predominate economic model is more than simply noticeable. Regulations have not worked and may have worsened the situation.

Somehow humans came to act as if they have a project on the planet. Humans like to own what they walk on and be mission oriented to claim that ownership. Projects are a means to fulfill missions and secure ownership. The most significant project of humans was driven by the idea of industry, via Newtonian science, and came to be centerpiece in defining human achievements. This is a human project with a purpose of stabilizing the meeting of human needs. Simultaneously this created a threat to natural systems and their stability. Via a Newtonian logic of rational analysis, mechanistic cause-effect logic, and homocentric domination humans developed in clear opposition to nature and the natural order that we once looked upon as ecosystems. We now see humans trying to redesign genetic codes to replicate natural design, all while working towards creating a system of artificial intelligence to control and manage natural systems and natural intelligence.

Is this good? Based on the experience of industrialization so far, we have reason to be concerned in this direction of development. Can it have a good ending? Are humans capable of managing all this around us since they have yet to manage themselves? What is nature's role in the making of the artificial process and in the longer-term prospects of life on earth? Does nature occupy another dimension in the universe, or is she only a struggling force in the third dimension to planet earth?

It's helpful to see how the human attitude to nature has evolved. Beginning in fright, then worship, then respect and finally to seeing nature as a servant to human use. Recently, some shame has surfaced in the human attitude towards nature. Some humans feel badly that humans turned nature into a depository for the backside of industrialization, where the deposits spread through the oceans, landscapes, and air. Soon the manly attitude towards nature may well have gone full circle and turned to fear.

There are early signs of a justified fear by humans of nature, in the human perception of her. She is increasingly recognized as supplying the essentials of life. Some humility is returning to humans yet the signs of acting no this are scant. How to state this in a more recognizable manner to humans? One means is to note how humans somehow relate closely to religious metaphors, especially when thinking of that which we do not understand. Thus, we might say humans have "desecrated nature" via industrialization and now might best fear retribution from nature. Moving beyond this, what is happening to the environment on which humans depend and what best might they do to deal with the consequences of past actions? Or is it simply too late to manage those consequences?

Even with signs of a human change on the horizon there is little indication that this change will bring a radical difference to our definition of the industrial. Computerization of the artificial will only further enhance its status with humans against the natural. We will still favor a 19th Century Newtonian paradigm of industrialization. It is hard for a human project to change the centerpiece of what defines that project. Industrialization has long supplied the goods desired by man and done so via a 19th Century paradigm of economics supplying human needs while marketing to its ever-expanding human wants. This seemingly guarantees continuation of business as usual even while the winds of a natural disaster approach. How best might humans respond, once they decide they must? Can we find a replacement for industrial, to Newton, to Smith, to economics and to rediscover the role of the natural of which we are a part?

The role of human activities, especially bio-needs turning to economic wants, was derived from how we met biological needs. That approach left deterioration to the natural in the wake of achievement of the artificial. If nature was found to be important later there surely was an artificial recipe to "fix things." What was once seen as implicitly manageable, via more industrialization, now appears as explicitly dangerous to all life.

Our current best definition for meeting human needs, then moving to ever expanding wants, has turned quite bad and is now irreversibly changing the context of viable life on earth. Perhaps there is time for humans to change their economic values and/or their systems of production, and consumption, and valuation of the results, considering rethinking the human project. The best advice for humans just now seems to be developing an appreciation of nature and the larger cosmic context of life and the forces creating it. Of course, humans do not need to do such. They can continue with a business-as-usual approach until the context as stage set will become the main actor in the human play. As such humans will witness dramatic change to the essential conditions of life.

This is the context for the thesis presented herein and the driving force behind the research on which it is based. Those I worked with in the research mentioned by 2030 the impact of human acts on the environment will end in consequences to life beyond human repair. Humans will then experience the consequences of failing to improve their historic conceptions of business as usual. The research posed questions about human-capability for designing a learning-based means to change prior to human-managed change becoming irrelevant. There is little evidence for this possibility. Can innovation via business as unusual become the new standard? Can humans find a way to lessen the values of contemporary industrialization and redefine their vision of future business success to include the well-being of nature? Perhaps not. Options to better meet human needs while redirecting human wants are very exciting, but no one is reaching to develop them. Even adding computerization is little more than digitization of business as usual, faster. The war of the artificial against the natural continues.

Socrates appeared to offer the last best hope on regulatory context in Greece, but we should note how he came to end his life in a regulation event demanding self-inflicted poison. Likewise, Lao Tzu in China of the day offered an optimistic alternative to the normal societal emphasis on stability via control as argued for via Confucius followers. Regulatory leadership embraced Confucian thinking, even if it was unacceptable by most citizens, in that it emphasized stability of what was, not what should be, via central control. Lao Tzu instead gave emphasize to the continuous role of the normative, the becoming of what ought to be.

In 15th Century France Joan of Arc offered humans a different pathway to finding widespread societal leadership and governance. Her actions were consistent with teachings of Socrates and Lao Tzu but came to an end at age nineteen when the religious leaders of the day tied her to a burning stake to reflect upon her open disregard of their regulations. These disharmonies continue to be a part of societal development. In the 1970's an America version of leadership pasted a law to reduce the consumption of scarce petroleum. There were stiff penalties as threats to any who would be caught driving faster than 55 mph. This proved as counterproductive as the legacy it was based on. Some months later it was seen that the average driving speed was then higher than before the threats were imposed.

Does history show social systems to be wrong in the idea of regulation, or having the wrong leadership with their ideas, laws, regulations, governance, and management? Such questions seem important as modern social systems as they face very serious consequences of the present on the future. Perhaps it's not the ideas of regulation that are at fault but the set of ideas at the center of motivating social systems. A central idea relates to the economics of short-term results achievement that will provide for human needs and wants. Meeting these needs and wants has somehow come to be a fundamental good of social systems. As such, ideas about regulation should not interrupt such economic workings but move into control what are called the externalities of the work. What happens if regulation is not able to control the approaching long-term consequences of humans having achieved an abundance of short-term results?

If industrialization is based on use of tremendous quantities of energy to provide tremendous quantities of goods to meet bio and psycho needs and wants, and the process of meeting those needs and wants becomes the cause of human death, what shall we do to "regulate" the problems thus created? It's not too late to raise this question but maybe it's too late to answer it. Let us hope the human project finds a way to do well and turn from seeking ends that will end badly.

The human project has progressed far since humans emerged from the cave, or so humans have been taught and have come to believe? Humans, as one-time cave occupants, found their way out as portrayed in Plato's "Allegory of the Cave," then found new means to better provide for their needs while expanding a human need to satisfy their wants. Unfortunately, they failed to emerge from the limitations of humans relating to each other and their environments as acquired in the cave. Put another way, humans did escape the 2-dimensional restricted on perceiving reality as shadow movement on the cave's walls. But they failed to lose their homage to or attraction of management via the confused clarity of simple-minded concepts of 1-dimensional polarization. Prisoners would sit in their entrapments and learn to pretend they knew reality. This setting provided the necessary and sufficient conditions for life and adherence to the reality of their limited experiences. Later in the human project would be known as culture where humans would accept harshly authoritarian governance to protect culture from change. Its pervasion and perversion were clearly illustrated in Plato's Cave via the sad experiences of any who left the cave and attempted to return to describe the bondage of those remaining in the cave.

The eternal dilemma of human relations to truth was seen in the behavior of those who would bring new knowledge back from the edges of reality to comment on the different reality of the cave. Leadership served as the protector of those left in the cave and the major impediment to their moving to a higher state of knowing. The power of governance and legitimation of regulation thus began and were further developed to instill and preserve the permanence of the culture of the cave. The idea of change as threatening and the governance that protected cave dwellers from it became major impediments to improvement of the human project. Both stood in the way of progression of the human project and the finding of differences that made a more relevant difference to improvement.

Most cave dwellers came to appreciate changelessness and its war on differences that could not be trusted. The leadership of a culture based on changelessness retains authority by pointing out that new differences were simply wrong, and perhaps evil. Interesting for the study of regulation as presented herein is how at the edges of known reality could necessarily see how the beliefs of the core were wrong, and often silly. Yes, those at the core of a culture, its leaders, and managers, would retain authority via this emphasis on differences out there that might be harmful, or negate the meaning of the culture. This included religions, governments, corporations, and even scientific disciplines. The study of regulations illustrates these cultural differences as well as the ominous nature of challenges facing humans in not turning to differences that made a good difference in dealing with bad differentials.

Back to Plato's Cave. Humans continue to accept the ideological strait jacket forms of 1-dimension regulation/leadership noted by Socrates in Plato's Cave. Humans continue to accept a 2-dimensional interpretation of reality as seen in the shadows on the cave ceiling via finding legitimation in writings on 2-dimensional paper that get interpreted by 1-dimensional judges. The notion of moving on to a 3-dimensional governance scheme of virtual managers remains a dream, or unimaginable. This is more than a problem of effectiveness in dealing with the 3-dimensional reality we occupy, but increasingly involves the largely unknown and much unappreciated 4-dimensional entropic reality that threatens three-dimensional life. Humans seem happily uninformed as they move into a crisis while carrying the consequences of their behavior in the 3rd dimension into the irreversible 4th dimension.

To be fair, a few of the "regulated prisoners" did escape the bondage of Plato's cave and did come to experience a 3-dimensional reality beyond their 2-dimensional "Flatland". From this the mental leader of Plato's Cave, Socrates, could sense pointlessness (A trait of the 0-dimension.) of continued 1-dimensional leadership in society based on religions not subject to questioning. Once outside the confines of the cave occupants could marvel at the nature represented by a sun passing through a 4-dimensional timeframe, although this vision made their eyes hurt and caused their minds to become confused. Two thousand years later humans would come to marvel at the 4-dimensional entropic movement of time in nature. While we now begin to see this entropic arrow of time as leading to our non-existence, we now cannot conceive of a 5th- dimensional reality surrounding the entropic passing of something into nothing.

As such, humans continue to occupy caves while making an environmental mess of life in the 3rd dimension as well as using economics to speed up 4th-dimensional entropy. This presents a potentially hopeless situation for the human future. Can human activities be regulated, or their consequences be otherwise resolved? This question grows louder with time and has greatly increased during the past two decades of the past two centuries. Underlying the emerging situation is a deeply seated human belief that nature furnishes humans with a storehouse of resources for human use. As such dimensional differences to the realities of the human project and largely ignored as is the wisdom lying in the 5th dimension, a wisdom that may well make humans irrelevant.

Humans came to feel free of biological needs and having to negotiate with nature over them. Humans could relax and not worry about their need for food, water, and shelter. Humans could avoid the historic feelings of terror towards natures' variations, vicissitudes, and violence. Humans could then move forward to build a homo-centric project on earth, and beyond, and move the human project from meeting needs to satisfying human wants. Human projects could be counted on to simply do better and better without end via human science and technology, without any meaningful restriction. Better and better than more could be the end in themselves. This could become the myth defining the meaningful human end state.

The research this is based on suggests a different sense of the context of humans, its condition, and its probable future for humans. Research carried out with the Petro-chemical industry and its governmental regulators suggests that what humans have done since leaving their caves may well have insured a dire future to the human project. Our best hope now seems to be returning to renegotiating with nature, but in a more ominous manner. Unlike life in the caves, restricted to seeing a 2-Dimensional flatland of images on a cave ceiling, the renegotiation needs to begin from a re-appreciation that there are important dimensions to life beyond the two of flatland. This includes the environmental dilemmas emerging in the 3rd-Dimension that call for knowledge from the context provided by an irreversible entropic 4th-Dimension. Since context matters to understanding we must do more to understand the context of the 4th-Dimenion; the nature of the 5th-Dimension and its meaning for humans. Just now our primary emphasis of on the economic potentials found in the third dimension, over which humans believe they have homocentric authority. Crucial to this control is the idea that humans can own and regulate property ownership. Most constitutions are drawn up with property ownership as a central tenant of regulation. This may make sense in the 3rd Dimension but lies between silly and becomes deadly in any 4th-Dimensional fast forward via limited wisdom of the homocentric. To survive, it seems that the human project needs to appreciate the context provided the 3rd Dimension by the movement of the 4th Dimension. As such the 4th Dimension requires appreciation of the 5th Dimension, whatever that may prove to be.

XII

LIFE'S DIMENSIONS,
IS THERE A 5th?

The sad potential in using traditional regulation in a new round of negotiation with nature is suggested herein. It will not be easy. More innovation is needed in the process. It will need to exceed the self-imposed restrictions humans have put on regulation via life in 2-Dimensions and its faith in what is written in a 2-Dimensional legal order. In it, humans have restricted the idea of potential harm to the strict logic found in 2 Dimensions. This is the domain West Churchman described as representing 10% of human reality. It is the same world taught in law school while depicted by Gregory Bateson as that which is within the sad limits of unaided rationality.

We start in the 2 Dimensions portrayed as reality as shadows for those restricted to Plato's cave. As such humans protect themselves from nature via manufacturing industrial-produced homes, manufactured consumer products, and industrialized agriculture as food. Humans can then concentrate on inventing new wants, needing new industrial products, and market ever more tangents of love. This process pretends stability yet portents crisis from the limitations of mechanized thinking leading to replacement of innate wisdom by seeking ever more intelligence of the artificial. This stimulates total arrogance ending in total ignorance. Is there a way out? is a way out necessary? How does nature relate to wisdom?

19th Century Industrialization thinking has become the potential for and the limitation of the human project. Is industrialization the best we can do? Is Newton's approach to industrialization as war on nature the best we can do? If humans remain a part of nature isn't this a war of humans against humanity. Is industrialization of the artificial the best we can do? If so, what is its end point? The model of industrialization criticized herein is from the stability hoped for in 19th Century Newtonian formulated presumptions guiding humans to see nature in a way so that we could control nature. The environmental deterioration results now pose considerable threats to life.

The tenants of Newton used herein begin in how 1) all effects can (even must) be traced back to their causes; then go on to argue how 2) force must be met with counter-force; 3) Euclid's Law of Parallels is fundamental (and it offers visual and static stability in designing an anti-natural, artificial environment); 4) success in human interactions (e.g., economics and other shared behaviors in pursuit of wants) is defined as the shortest distance between two points being a straight line (i.e., Adam Smith); 5) all things are understandable as a hierarchical structure (Herbert Simon's basis for receiving a 1978 Nobel Prize for the economics of Bounded Rationality and his argument for Artificial Intelligence.); and 6) life is neg-entropy (where action in a cesspool exemplifies the potentials in finding negative entropy in crating life as seen in Prigogine's 1977 basis for non-equilibrium thermodynamics and the basis for his Nobel Prize).

These Newtonian ideas operate in the zeroth, first and second dimensions of humanly defined realities. An argument will be presented, based on data from a two-year study of efforts to regulate the Petro-chemical industry, that we need to find a management doorway into the third dimension via an appreciation of the arrow that defines the fourth dimension and then the appreciate the humility necessary to sense a yet to be described fifth dimension, as therein lies the hope of negotiation with the forces of nature. This agenda is as challenging as it seems to be essential to the species.

DAVID HAWK

1. The Human Project, Towards A Fifth Dimension

Accepting that a human project is underway on the planet dare we ask if it has a mission, or even a discussable direction? Yes, religious and science bibles, such as Darwin's, suggest a purpose and direction for the species but besides using nature and/or researching nature what is the end point? While references these works are not the subject here. Herein we concentrate on the challenges in our utilization of natural resources to meet basic human needs and then evolve to feeling better by realization of the economics of human wants. This is not about economics or finance but the basic industrial processes that economists try to manage without understanding then fall back on finance to fill the gaps is our subject. Just now these are the limiting dimensions to human life on the planet. Finally, how does the human project get beyond these limitations and their consequences?

The ideas that structure our current reality come from a rational tool kit organized around a technological logic, a logic steeped in Newton's cause-effect thinking via Newtonian metaphors cloaked in the ignorance of nature. Behind this you can see a religious attitude encouraging nature's desecration. During the past two-hundred years of an industrial revolution we see technological development given almost complete credit for the advancement of societal affairs. Industrialization of the means of shelter building, food production, transportation and living has become the essence of the human project and its purpose. Crucial to this transformation has been the development of the sciences of the artificial. Imaging the artificial in defining and realization the mechanical has led to the fruits of industrialization, while heightening the war on nature. There is now discussion of the robotization of the human body to follow the mechanization and rationalization of the human mind.

All this had been derived from a continuous accessing of nature's stores of materials for product making, including houses, autos and connecting infrastructures. This is accompanied by ever expanded access to the energy required to make and use the products sought by human needs then human wants. More recently there has been an industrialization of agriculture. All this tends to refine as well as more deeply instill the values behind societies as well as how best to define human existence. All this was done to protect humans from the precariousness of nature via stabilizing natural change.

At the center of industrialization is the human project accessing, refining then consumption of Petro-chemicals. The Petro-chemical industry is at the center of the research on which the thesis described herein is based. It has made Petro-chemicals widely available to society in its development of the human project. In addition, it has recently come to be seen as a centerpiece in human efforts to regulate the cost to nature (i.e., externalities) of having and using these critical fuels of industrialization.

Humans recently began to be aware of unforeseen consequences to gains to the human condition from industrialization. Humans now begin to see consequences to extensive and expanding uses of Petro-chemicals in what we begin to note is environmental deterioration. The benefits of industrialization now appear to have costs as we see significant changes to environmental systems on which life, including human life, depends. This business-as-usual driving the human project is now beginning to be potentially dangerous to nature and thereby life which humans continue to have a stake in, regardless of emphasizing and greatly expanding the artificial. As such, humans are now expanding the role of regulation of the industry and its products. One subject of regulation, to reduce the unwanted, has been the Petro-chemical industry. The research reported herein focuses on the aspirations, successes, and failures of such societal regulation efforts. As will be outlined in some detail, the role of American trained lawyers in the success and failure of American attempt at regulation is critical to understanding failure. As Will Rogers said decades before: "The minute you read something you don't understand, you can be almost sure it was drawn up by a lawyer." In response the director of environmental concern regulation in another country commented on the 10,000-page USA Water Quality Act and attachments by saying: "We seem peculiar when compared to American lawyers. We believe the basis for a citizen to obey the law is to understand the law. Therefore, all environmental laws in our nation are written on twenty-five pages."

Social systems offer the subject herein. These include nation-states, cities, communities of interests, religions, cultures, political groups, companies, schools, and families. The emphasis here is on governmental and corporate systems that negotiate via regulations concerned with consequences of environmental deterioration and its trajectory for the planet.

Much attention is focused on social organizations negotiating over the future conditions of life, but an argument is made herein that the individual actor offers much insight and energy for the discussions, especially as society realizes more the limits to social regulation. Individuals are the basic element of social organizations as well as the source of independent thought and creativity for trying something new when the old fails. When business as usual begins to break down individuals generate the potential found in business as unusual.

The role of the individual is crucial to improving what an organization does when its performance reaches its limits, then breaks down when the context becomes intolerant of its behavior. When an organization reaches its limits, it turns to individuals for repair. An early systems scientist, Andras Angyal, noted that when a system reaches its limits, the parts assume the whole. This is noteworthy in that some contemporary social systems seem to be approaching or at their limits. Organizational limits are herein defined by their relations with and to a context. In the research this thesis is based on context is essential to determining limits.

Since industrialization humans generally turn to regulations for solving problems of systems. This generally involves discussion, notes of effects, speculating on cause(s), marking a possible path to solution, then drawing of written laws or rules to manage the detected cause. For example, if too many citizens are seen to be consuming too many mind-altering drugs, then laws against their use will be drawn up. Of course, this will exclude the drugs designed and distributed by major drug companies then prescribed to patients by licensed doctors. Only when the first stage fails do humans look at the much larger activities of the drug companies and the doctors they are related to.

One consequence, not considered at the beginning of the regulation, is that the process of governance of drug use will be less than successful thus requiring expansion of prisons to house those who fail to obey the regulation as promulgated. Where a forbidden drug intersects with prescribed drugs the legal process will attempt ignore those said to be legal. To do otherwise makes the legal process unworkable. This model of regulation is largely derived from a Newtonian model of reality and use of its metaphors. Newtonian thinking and Newtonian based regulation is mostly restricted to 2-dimensional imaging that derives its legitimacy from laws as written and emphasizes the 1-dimension that points to the law as written.

Humans sometime raise their eyes and make use of a larger set of resources available in 3-dimensional reality. While it is exceedingly rare, some humans (not those trained to be lawyers) even reflect on the impact of regulation in the 4th-dimension. This is the domain of the longer-term consequences of environmental deterioration. Those who find the 3rd dimension available to them often resolve their problem in need of regulation by moving to another location. Many who begin to experience the consequences of a problem misuse the 4th dimension to away a solution or see the problem float away. A few seek solutions beyond cause-effect by looking into the 4th dimension. Based on the research behind this writing there is reason to believe that the more legitimate solutions of problems of consequence are in appreciate of the 5th dimension. To date science cannot find this dimension. It is where there is understanding of the 2nd Law of Thermodynamics as seen to define the 3rd dimension, i.e., that gives time its arrow. Herein most discussion will focus on regulation activities generated in the 1st dimension and implemented in the 2nd dimension, with some 3rd dimensional conclusions suggested.

This document mostly ignores those operating from the pointlessness of the 0th dimension, although some examples of their problem-solving capabilities are given. One is where the state of New York tested many wells on Long Island and found them all polluted and in need of repair. Since there was no known repair at an affordable cost the regulatory issue was resolved via removing the funds for further testing of wells. A similar result came from a New Jersey law saying toxic wastes could not exist in the state.

On occasion, humans face phenomena beyond the capabilities of laws as written, movement in space, and movement in time. This calls for imagining of the 5th dimension of reality, a place human imaging, even imagination, is ill-equipped to enter. This may become important to realize in face of the most ominous situations facing life and living. In this domain the idea of regulation seems trivial, as does the capabilities of governance. As such, other kinds of human conceptualization are required. Needed innovation often begins outside the social system, at the level of the individuals. Social systems tend to favor stability and thus prefer changelessness more than individuals. Throughout human history individuals arise from the organization to propose unorthodox ideas. These individuals are later called leaders but even the idea of a leader being able to resolve an ominous situation may now be diminished. Leadership is now mostly associated with entertainment and/or wealth, and not management of crisis.

Societal leaders often create chaos, not resolve it. Thus, humans may want to go light on awaiting leaders to resolve serious social problems. Herein we will not turn against the idea of leaders resolving environmental challenges but will see individuals as those, when stimulated, can generate ideas on improvement that a total system does not.

Individuals are essential parts to an organization yet are viewed as suspect by that same social organization. Those emphasizing the maintenance of an organization worry about those who talk of reconstructing the organization or suggesting they will simply leave it and initiate a new organization. As such the social group is always concerned about what some individuals are up to. This can be seen in how the first group makes use of the latest technology to covertly monitor the second group while the second group uses the same technology to openly communicate with the total organization. When change is needed in regulation this distinction will be important. Opponents to regulation are often seen as anarchists. This is not helpful, nor accurate.

2. Nature as the Ultimate Regulator

Relying on dimensional locations does little to resolve previously initiated difficulties inherent to the consequences of climate change. The shortcomings in 0 through the 3rd dimensionality, as outlined previously, are mostly dealt with via an entropic death within the 4th dimension, but such removes life from the situation. As termination that is a serious problem form. Entropy manages that 4th dimension. We should remember that this moves into the domain of the non-rational and raises questions, such as is it more negative entropy, but also opens up hope in that it exists outside rational description thus enters the edges of what we call physical sciences as in cutting edge physics.

The distinction between "lawful" and "legal." You cannot find or create a process of negative entropy, via the laws of thermodynamics, but it is legal for you to market such then when needed legally argue that it might not be real, but you were, are, will, would or could be.

Humans, where their anger over Entropy becomes a major addition to the Entropic Process. Since there is seldom meaning without a context for a statement you might look at the math of A^4 passing through D^4 (4 dimensions of 4 stages of our context). Keep in mind this all unfolds within the 5th dimension. Without context there cannot be meaning where meaning is the basis for everything. As such the hierarchies and the power, they imply but do not give are irrelevant. Concentrating on cause-effect thinking can provide knowledge that encourages hierarchies. Standing back to watch the effects of effects on context gives access to the wisdom essential to life's continuance.

END STATE OF STRATETIC BEINGS:

- Human Attitude: To Denigrate
- Strategic Human Actions: To Deteriorate
- Results: Denial
- Contextual Consequences: Death

Isn't it great to be a member of humankind? It's like traveling in an arrogance-filled balloon seeking intent from the content. We descend into misunderstanding life while shopping for what we don't need, like or what.

3. Continuing the Search for Who We Are

Earlier in the book "negative entropy" was introduced as crucial to the manly attitude of arrogance over nature. "Whatever the problem, we will find our way out from it, usually via new technology." These days it is again in the news relative to producing energy with no cost and conducting it with no loss.

It helps us to understand who we are and from where our human limits arise. You may not enjoy this, but neg-entropy could come to be the most significant symbol of humans seeking meaning and thus inventing bullshit to drive human development. Neg-entropy would be sold as a driver of change, yet its impossibility insures changelessness. It was key to the religions developed prior to the industrial. It then became a sacred idea at the center of the ideas that created the design of the industrialization pathway humans chose. Via it we built an interstate highway into the 6th extinction of life via climate change.

Climate change consequences offer us an introduction to the early results of humanly created environmental deterioration. Humans are said to be becoming scared, yet recent studies released by George Mason and Yale show how only 15% of Americans feel climate change will lead to "a great deal of personal harm." 33% believe that such will affect future generations and the poor, not them. People having trouble finding clean drinking water or floating away on car roofs in floods live elsewhere. Reasons for concern are off in the far distant future. Meanwhile, they look out their window in pride at the magnificence of the huge SUV they just bought, to show neighbors the magnificence of the owner. They do not feel as if they are or soon will be fucked, in the awful, non-sexual, sense of the concept. *Herein, to feel fucked is a notation that a life-changing experience is approaching and will take you in a negative direction.* This differs from losing your job, so you are thus available for a better job, or losing a spouse you love who believes meanness is a good doorway to improving self-importance.

You need to try to recover from bipolar arguments around you that are intended to support political leadership that expresses: "Making America Great Again." Parents accept such bullshit as the price of entry from which there ends up being no exit. The 20th Century expanded use of clarification terms such as fuck was to reveal the historic role of diminishing the lower, poorer classes by banning their use of certain terms and avoiding they use in speaking truth to power by telling management to "fuck off" with their idiot orders and exaggerated salaries. You can see how this was changed in the fifties and sixties by such greats as Lenny Bruce and George Carlin. If you would like, please go back to the longer history of the 16th to 21st Centuries articulation of being fucked as will be outlined in the book.

It's enough for now to reflect on "fuck you" as a stay away warning to someone being strategic in their behavior, as distinct from open, honest, and concerned for your wellbeing. Being strategic is something like a parent, spouse, lawyer, policeman, politician, and boss asking you questions to try finding out those things that you have reason to not tell them. You know what I mean, everyone does.

Most humans see the forthcoming bad as only temporary. They point out that the climate is always changing, that is its definition. Time brings good and bad to visit us, but as we will become immortal why worry about the details of life. 95% of scientists see the future as catastrophic to continuance of life. That optimistic 5% studied Human Resources and Marketing in a business program tailored (Frederic Taylor) on Harvard's truths.

Where lies the future, in human change or continuation of lies? Climate is changing in ways that cannot become reversed for thousands if not millions of years depending on whether the global temperature rises 2- or 5-degrees C. Optimism is a trait of leaders we seek so why not see the "glass as half full, not half empty"? From my research since 1975 it's clear the glass is actually empty and covered in urine stains. Thus, a debate is now emerging in much of our world: "are we fucked?" My work found this debatable in 1975. In 2025 the work of many others now sees the situation as "too late."

Humans that are concerned about the shadows endeavor to find a clear cause for the shadow effect. This has become the pattern via the worship of the industry as based on continual development of science and technology. This replaced their prior worship of an angry god displeased human behavior. Just now humans are coming to place their trust in political processes that provide leadership confined to consistently turning right at all intersections, or a consistent left at the same decision points about their future.

Some humans would like to argue that the transformation comes from a footnote Darwin left out, or a chapter that Karl Marx and/or Adam Smith included. In fact such changes are not well understood by traditional *cause-effect* thinking of scientists wanting to own, patten and profit from their truths. Another method is required to see the more systemic interactions of groups of relations upon an active context. Herein we will call this the *effects-from-effects*, i.e., future effects as derived from prior effects.

Therein we see contemporary effects arise from effects of prior extensive development, i.e., the capturing and organization of extensive materials and energy from the context to meet what humans claim as their bio-needs and psycho-wants. Such a process was depicted in the 2021 movie advising humans to avoid "Looking Up." That "Don't Look Up" movie commandment depicted humans as fucked and thus acting to fuck up their planet via choices of leadership via ideas and/or bodies on two legs with nowhere to go. Such came to be seen to unfold as leadershit of contemporary society not leadership of ancient dreams. Historically leadership was mostly concerned with the collective called others. Leadershit may begin with such ideas but soon concentrate on the power of selfishness seen at the core of self.

Humans are now watching a rerun of the movie but differently in than humans are directly responsible for the harm coming to them and their planet, not a random meteor that arrives from the cosmos. Some, mostly scientists, see how human valuing gains to self over all others comes to be responsible for the impending problem. This value accomplishes much in the short term, but as we can now see, it presents great costs in the longer term. The current effects of prior efforts to effectively provide for bio-needs and psycho-wants are being seen in effects from droughts, floods, and rising temperatures in landscapes and oceans. The context of stability required for life on earth is becoming greatly disrupted and sent into motion, much like the Emery and Trist paper of 1965 described as turbulence.[103] In 1975 I had suggested that Trist add a Type V context to depict conditions of climate change, to be called the "black hole" of the 21st Century. He was my key advisor on the dissertation subject that this book draws on.

Humans are the force of destruction of our context, and not a random meteor that appears from the cosmos. In the 2021 movie where you are advised "to not look" and simply accept there is little you can do and if you want your closing moments on earth to be happy then just smile. In our current reality of 2024 you are advised to not "wake up" as such will be disruptive to our political and economic systems reality. The quiet advice from our news and most websites is that even if you have ideas for un-fucking the disasters from our future its best to remain silently "un-awake."

---

[103] Emery and Trist, "The causal texture of organizational environments," London: *Humans Relations*, 18(1) 21-32, 1965.

XIII

TOO LATE FOR REGULATORS

1. Can Humans Regulate Themselves?

Organizations continually fear their individuals will move into an anarchistic posture, in the French American sense of the term, where chaos is the consequence. Who knows, individuals might destroy the organizational core. They stored capital wealth would thus be disassembled. This sense of anarchy is opposite to the sense originally given by Greek philosophers. Therein it was the individual being co-managed in partnership with nature, as in "the sailboat without rudder." The individual, as anarchist, thought to be an early warning system stationed at the edge of social organizations, would inform the whole of a need to change. Individuals like Socrates, P. Kropotkin, and M.L. King illustrate the importance of such.

But there are major dichotomies between social systems and their semi-independent members. It is important to understand these to then understand the dilemmas in social regulation. The difference between the social group and the individual is fundamental to understanding larger issues of governance and where and why they turn to regulation as a tool for problem control. This is just now important as we may be encountering a problem that is not open to regulation or governance. Perhaps only individual appreciation of the problem and their personal role in it can unravel it.

To lower the suspicion of the social system towards the individual members individuals pass through public educated to learn to be subservient to the social group. This is seen as important to the functioning of social organizations. Individuals are often seen as capable of objecting to the social group and are thus a target for social intimidation. Regulation is the dominant means of control. Some individuals are potential anarchists, i.e., as threats to operations of the group. As such, they need to be carefully watched, some must even be imprisoned. Socrates, P. Kropotkin, and M. L. King illustrate the essence of the problem posed to a social system by an intelligent and highly moral individual, especially in an immoral society. Such individuals operate at the edge of the social system, and never in its core. Sometimes a system moves to embrace the thinking at the edge to survive but even then, the anarchist stays at the edges. Such people are essential to a social system that needs ominous change and on occasion the human project requires very drastic movement.

Why is this in an introduction to research into regulation of environmental deterioration? As deterioration expands from an acceptance of environmental desecration and the consequences therein the dangers become more three-dimensional and noticeable. Just now we begin to see signs of change in four dimensions. A new form of response to this seems urgent. At the root of all this is a deeply held belief in ever expanding industrialization, and expansion of the artificial via it. Such expands on the war against nature. The end of such is to serve human needs ever more in attempts to satisfy human wants, herein called psycho-wants. The widespread acceptance of a need to desecrate the natural ends in deterioration via pollution and the unwanted being dumped in the larger environment.

The way out will involve a critic of societal acceptance of desecration. This will involve an appreciation of human-nature relations and rethinking the cost of industrialization. This is best done at the individual level as worker, employee, consumer, shopper, and citizen. As individuals like M.L. King have illustrated, the societal context is slow to appreciate what is obvious to the individual. Evidence from the research behind this work shows how innovation and improvement is best seen and implemented by individuals, especially those at the edge. Expanding society regulation seems to only worsen a situation in need of change. This change is seen in the consequences of industrialization. The interest behind this paper is with where lies the power directing humans to do what they do, and how can that power be managed to do better?

We have two major options for the regulator to consider. Is the activity designed to manage the bad or to encourage the good? The difference in attitude is significant relative to results, as shown in the Stockholm study. The first option gives societal leadership the right to make society more civil by emphasizing the wrong and making it righter. The second option reverses the targets and gives emphasis to the doing of good. Emphasis of the first is with punishment of those doing wrong, unless they have the power to publicly define bad as good because they only do good. Management in the second option is different. Therein few would be locked up and the economic sector of managing prisoners would be bankrupt.

Society often elects option a) to avoid significant change, even when it is widely felt that society itself is bad. This is like changing oil in a car that ought not to be on the road. If the guiding principles of a society emphasize the doing of what comes to be bad, then can there be much hope for use of regulation to change their values to force them to do good? Probably not. Doing the good while avoiding the doing of the bad will be profound to any continuation of life on the planet, or so the research results on which this writing is based imply.

In simple terms, the continuation of life on this planet is based on the actions of humans while they live on the planet. Humans now emphasize strategic management in that they have come to believe longer-term strategies are more powerful than results achievement in the present. In that the definer of strategic thinking argued that strategy is deceitful and to be successful with strategy one must not be transparent of honest then this thinking may simply bring higher dangers to the long term. It would seem humans need to replace the strategic management that replaced results management with consequential management. Those actions have consequences. Herein the results of human actions come with aspects of environmental deterioration where the processes surrounding environmental deterioration have consequences beyond the intended results. These are mostly referred to as "unintended" consequences, not because they are not known but they are mostly ignored and said to simply be "the price of progress" for the human project. Perhaps we can look closer at the definition given to progress prior to perhaps clarifying the sinister end to the human project, and humans?

It is unclear how to best accomplish the first, to encourage the good in humans. Most societies introduced religious forms to use as a vehicle to argue for and expand on the good side of mankind. As such humans are attracted, temporarily, to preachers and teachers. Follows then tap into their predisposed feelings of use the atmosphere of the good as an ideal camouflage to cover their practicing of the bad.

The good is generally outside and above religious precepts and education forms. We are best served to not give too much credit or blame to the cultures of religious beliefs and educational norms. Both domains tend to be abstracted from meaningful realities. They seldom relate to the good or the bad. Thus we wander between the good and bad with no reference to the consequences of each and both. This weakness is fundamental to shortcomings in the world of governance, of regulation, and of leadership. Much more can be said about this world, then asked of it. As such learning more of regulation requires addressing questions such as:

1) What regulation is?
2) Are there different models of how to regulate?
3) Are those that emphasize force upon the bad, to do good, more successful than those that try to encourage all to do better?
4) Are those educated in law suitable to both approaches, and only the first?
5) Can regulation worsen what it works to improve?

2. Context: The Ultimate Regulator

This writing is derived from a relatively large two-year study done at the Stockholm School of Economics into best means to reverse environmental deterioration that ended with evidence that there were no known means and the consequences for the planet would be severe. Regulation of social systems was the emphasis in that two-year study and will be the focus herein but presented in a way that is less optimistic than the beginning of the study. Global warming, acidification of rain, changing climate conditions, plasticizing of the oceans, etc. offer no reason of optimism in the consequences of human behavior.

Concern herein is with attempts to regulate societal systems to enhance the societal good and reduce the bad. This is a heavy agenda, often done badly and generally directed at individuals seen to be not doing good by societal definition, those of other races, religions, or low incomes. Such individuals via regulation are coerced, threatened, or simply forced to change their behavior via trivial to serious penalties on their lives. Those who write such laws then set up means and methods to enforce them are at the center of the process. The process has many names but herein we shall call it "legalism." This comes from those at the center being trained in the profession called lawyers.

Our central question herein is: how successful can legalism be in "forcing" individuals to behave in ways that are in opposition to what their culture has trained them to do and be? If teenagers have been taught that they are breaking some unimportant law by drinking and driving, but it's sort of okay if they are careful, drive slowly and don't get caught, or are stopped by an enforcer that is a former classmate, much like happens to their parents, then what is the social harm? Viewed in another way, what then is the value of legalism except to gainfully employ lawyers, where the United States has about five times as many per capital as its trading partners? Then, we might ask which is a stronger regulator of behavior, laws as written and enforced by narrow professionals or cultural behaviors that are widely acceptable in and used to define the culture?

Where the law, as written by lawyers, is unsuccessful are there alternative modes that can work better? Ought they be written by non-lawyers as happens in some other countries, or is there unwritten regulation that works better? Or is the best hope to practice good for society come from change to the culture and its definition of good?

The next deeper question then becomes: If a set of cultural ideas provides the economic goods and services necessary to a society and goes deeper to define societal success in wants ownership can it be changed? This begins in a perception of what is socially desirable and undesirable, and then how this viewpoint thus relates to any definitions of good/bad in a context seen as relevant, perhaps even meaningful. Context is thus crucial to regulation effectiveness in that it is basic to all evaluation.

There is much yet to be known about context and its emerging growth in importance. A few scientists have noted that context seems in motion and with time the movement is becoming more rapid and less predictable. Using time, space or prediction of cycles can no longer keep necessary stability in human context. That work of Emery and Trist in the mid-sixties set the foundation for what is now accepted as a genuine concern for societies. Thinking of our surroundings as a stage set for human acting Emery and Trist suggested that the stage set would increasingly become the subject of the play, not the human actors.

Before concentrating on environments and their emerging turbulence we need to see the variations available to any who analyze: 1) the desirable/undesirable, 2) the good/bad, and 3) the right/wrong. All three have a relationship to cultural world of the artificial but a bio-physical link to the world of nature becomes more noticeable with time. As such we need to improve our ways of including differences in values, morals and operations in are study of regulation methods but not in their segmented analytic sense. They need to be viewed as whole with the parts systemically connected as a network of operations, not a hierarchy. Appreciation must cut across all three not set up in isolation so each can seem to contradict the others.

Legalism often relies on this approach as well as adding other methods of ambiguity.

Ambiguity in what is written and what is adjudicated can become crucial to allow the good and right to be undesirable. Analysis via segmentation and reductionism are helpful to future ambiguity, especially where it is used to obscure an ominous event that is approaching. This insight is helpful to see much of what is addressed in this work, but it may raise questions irresolvable by humans.

For shorthand purposes let's assume desirable activities are those seeming to enhance life, while the undesirable seems to denigrate life, and the living. The deeper problem dealt with herein comes from evidence that recent regulation activities set up to control fundamental relations between man and nature, relations growing more dangerous to life with time, are not working.

The distinction between the good and bad is of course important but will only be referenced herein as a doorway into the darkness posed in Goethe's Faustian Struggle, a battle that says much about the challenges to and limitations of societal regulation. This is where humans generally seek short-term promises while ignoring the long-term consequences of having realized those promises. More poetically, this is the long-standing human fantasy of concentrating on work for short-term rewards while hoping the long-term costs will evaporate, be resolved by new technology, or pass on to unmet or unknown others. For example, via industrialization and extensive use of energy and materials to gain products for human needs it is widely known that there will be and are long-term consequences. This piles-up as environmental deterioration and as they pile up more, and are more ignored, they lead humans into a culture of environmental desecration. This desecration becomes central to an economic process where we alter resources taken from nature for products essential to human needs for food, shelter, and security, and then expand on the process to satisfy human wants. In more scientific short form this is where we create products for now via our ideas of negative entropy while rapidly expanding entropy's arrow into the future.

This provides a context for the work presented herein where the work focuses on explicit then implicit difficulties in regulating human dilemmas in their search for the good and bad, then seek ways to govern the differences. Central to the governance as it is now practiced are laws that are written and quickly adjudicated, then abdicated. The record of success in solving problems via regulation is questionable at best, nonsensical on average, and deadly at worse. Unjust laws, written with analytic precision about small parts of very large wholes can lead to problems larger than those initiated by the laws. They can lead to warfare, as well as an uninhabitable context for life.

Interest is with regulation efforts to manage individual activities to induce the species to do well by doing the good. At the center of this is the question can humans be effectively managed if they have free will, or belief in expressing it? Or is free will the key to individuals rethinking who and what they are in breaking away from the idea of "follow the leader" no matter how mistaken he is? Regulation, is viewed herein, is seen as a human response to a challenge arising from leadership that has led wrongly and governed mistakenly. This is especially apparent where regulation is based on laws written in an esoteric manner by people trained in law schools to pretend what they cannot know to protect the community that does not understand. This was clearly illustrated in some American refineries in a non-American location that were far cleaner than the same kind of refinery was in America. In America the water quality laws and attachments were written on ten thousand pages. In the other country all environmental laws, including water quality, were written on twenty-five pages. The success in reducing environmental deterioration in that country was remarkable. When asked, the Head of environmental quality in that country was asked why they restricted their laws to twenty-five pages. His response: "We are funny about regulations. We believe the first stop to obeying a law is to understand it." His American counterparts were upset with this response they called "naive." The dilemma for the Americans so commenting was that the later results in the non-American facilities were far better than what the Americans felt to be "sophisticated".

Special emphasis is herein on an emerging class of relationship difficulties that appear beyond human methods of control. Current definitions of leadership seem incapable of adequately describing the difficulties except to say they seem to arise from nature and might have been initiated by industrial activities. Humans are gradually accepting that the difficulties pose a danger to systems of life but in the longer term. Many describe such difficulties as being complex but are being worked on to make them understood. This depiction seems unhelpful in that the research explicitly seeks to describe the effects then move to the causes. Seldom are they discussed as systemic difficulties. Complexity is often in the eye of the beholder, and not intrinsic to a lightly understood systemic subject. When we posit that our relationship to another human is complicated, we usually mean he/she is wrong, but we don't want to say so. We imply that the relation contains a network of culturally incompatible issues that we avoid unraveling, as we know of no solution therein. It may be the same in human-nature relations in that we fear the economic consequences of no longer seeing nature as a storehouse of resources for our willful use, or a dumping ground for that which humans have used.

The class of these challenging relations includes how humans have related to nature and then, how nature is redefining her relations to humans. Humans have long ignored nature via a culture defined by industrialization. This did not involve complexity but did involve ignorance based on past cultural beliefs from such wisdom as that suggested in biblical advice such as: "go forth and use offered resources." Now humans meet the consequential feedback from nature, but with no known means to manage the consequences from the human environment. Research behind this thesis shows regulations applied to this problem area were someplace between ineffective and exacerbating of the challenge to find resolution.

Relations can always be "complicated," even complex, but this mostly implies the relations in question are outside the current capability to understand them. In some instances, this can be explained as a viewer desiring to see an analytically stable hierarchy instead of seeing a systemically organized network in constant change. This is not a criticism of colleagues but a suggestion we carefully consider Gregory Bateson's depiction of a limitation built into modern human thinking. This is the limited thinking process he titled: "unaided rationality."

There is a more reflective process that seems to emerge in youth, those pre-teens that sense the arrival of a new pattern of relations. It is as if they come from another world, not one that humans own as their human project via a contemporary culture of knowing what is and isn't reality. The emphasis on rational meaning as sent to us in thoughts of Confucius, Plato, Kant, et.al., now seem insufficient to the challenges of emerging relationships of the systems we occupy. As such, regulations are a doorway into another place, not the means to control the place we now believe we occupy. Most human endeavors, such as attempts at regulation, must be based on learning at various levels. Bateson's model as paraphrased in Figure 2.1 shows its importance.

There are many categories of relations involving humans. Some are between humans and humans, often labeled the social. Others are seen to exist between humans and nature where previously the relation was battle between humans and nature, where we look on it with pride as the industrial was destined to release humans from the needs given us by nature. Now, with less pride over time, some humans note that the relationship was a Faustian Bargain of the long-term payment for some short-term gains. The gains were freedom from needs, access to fulfilling wants and the human project headed towards happiness. The longer-term consequences were environmental pollution and deterioration that would close the entire human-nature relation. A third relationship is becoming as disheartening as the second. It is where humans as individuals confront themselves, their nature, their own character and what it means. Even with the aid of shopping, drugs, and entertainment the meaning is largely found insufficient. This is the world of the psychological.

3. From Education to Learning, The "Questions"

Regulation is supposed to resolve problems between things. There are laws against humans hurting each other, except maybe for few restrictions on use of guns, and laws against environmental pollution being put in nature and some drugs put into humans. Closer examination shows serious shortcomings in this process of regulation. For example, in 1972 it was agreed in the US that there was a serious problem in pollution passing into water systems from industrial production facilities. The laws were primarily written by Senator Muskie and his staffers. When they all were interviewed they pointed out that: "Sure we knew there were problems in the National Water Quality Act we drew up, but we decided to simply get something out three to deal with problem, then in a " year or two drag it back in and fix it based on knowing more about it." This seems okay, except in 1978 we still await its "suitable repair." Except for sending industrial facilities to other countries little has been accomplished in water quality improvement, or even stabilization.

There are many problems within and between these categories with some of them very serious, even deadly. Humans often resort to regulations out of fear of consequences from problems, simply to get hold of the problems as they see them. The general objective is to stabilize the context needed for life, i.e., to gain back control of that which seems to control the human project as it is contemporaneously defined. This process is not necessarily bad but if it is designed via analysis, as based on analysis, and deemed analytically beneficial it leads to deeper instability and hopelessness. In the research that the thesis herein is based on the following example was found. In the early seventies water pollution was found to be a significant threat to life and human well-being. The Environmental Water Quality Act was framed passed and implemented. Senator Muskie and his staffers were central writers of the Act. When interviewed he and his staffers argued: "Sure, we know it is not the solution for water pollution now occurring, but we want to just get something out there to see how it works and then drag it back in and repair it in a year or two when we know more" of how to do it. It awaits repair.

Much evidence for success/failure of regulation can be gained for the three areas via inquiring into the relations between humans and their artificially constructed environments. These include the industrial framework within which most humans live and define their success in life. It certainly includes the industrial plants and energy organizing facilities on which the industrial project depends, but also includes the organization of products from those plants and the energy use such projects require. This includes enlightened design of man-made environments to inspire independence within collective forms of social organization. It also includes the attempts at regulations in all the above, including building materials laws and their enforcement. Relative to the thesis mentioned in the opening we even see problems in governance of that which humans understand or should understand since they created it. Instructive of this point US Supreme Court cases on building products regulations. They conclude in their review of this area this is the most corrupt area of regulations they have seen. Perhaps they say this about all areas they study? Regardless, please take note that there are serious problems in laws, regulations, and governance everywhere. Many of these come from the limited knowledge of the legal professionals trained to manage such as abstractions. This is not what is covered in this document. The concern here is with emergent issues that are not appreciated, not those issues of judicial conflict as humans have come to understand the role of regulation in the human project.

Humans take greatest pride in that which rises above the limitations and restrictions of nature as they perceive nature. While also being part of nature humans seem to be working on a project to control and even eliminate nature. There is a growing reliance on this as relations between humans and their artificial environments, especially the computerization of human activities. Surely regulation will be applied in these areas of human relationships and their governance.

Difficulties in relations can be depicted in various ways but generally rely on economic, political, judicial, and personal terminology applied within and/or between the subject areas. Most recently, difficulties in human relations with the natural environment have emerged in human consciousness as of potential importance although presumed to be less important than economic relations. During times of drastic societal conflict, e.g., wartime, the emphasis is with man-to-man relations. After war the emphasis moves to the consequences of that war and attention centers on the psychological and then its relation to the ethical. As the consequences of man-nature relations become more apparent this area of difficulty is likely to be more a focus and a greater target for resolution via regulations.

The Stockholm project found use of the concept of learning was crucial to change regulations, thus keeping the process as fluid as the phenomena being regulated. This is the model of learning used in that project to ensure change was part of it, not court room arguments about avoiding change.

> **Zero learning** - No learning takes place here. The activity is characterized by simple and direct responses, which, regardless of whether they are right or wrong, are not subject to any change or correction. (For example, there is a command-and-control simplicity, where hierarchical orders are given and taken without question.)

> **Level 1. learning** - This is change in aspects of specific responses. Correcting errors of choice is allowed, but only within a narrow range of alternatives. (For example, alternatives to a set of project specifications are allowed, or given.)

> **Level 2. learning** - This is a change in the process of Level I; such as making a corrective change in the set of alternatives from which a choice is made or change in how the sequence of experiences are punctuated. (For example, there is a moving between assignments, or learning to do a variety of jobs)

> **Level 3. learning** - is change in the process of Level II, e.g., a corrective change in the system of sets of alternatives from which choice is made. (We shall see later that to demand this level of performance of some men and some mammals is sometimes pathogenic. This could involve redefining the sexual habits of men in a protestant community, or to have

those building nuclear power stations to switch to photo-voltaic stations.)

Level 4. learning - is a change in Level III, but probably does not occur in any adult living organism on this earth. The evolutionary process has, however, created organisms whose ontogeny brings them to Level III. The combination of phylogenesis with ontogenesis, in fact, achieves Level IV. (This would involve people learning not to go to war, to achieve a new relationship to nature.)

Level 5. Learning – Only occurs within the 5th dimension of non-existence as described elsewhere.

4. Four Domains for Categorizing Humans

Langer's comments give insight to two ideas, both of which we encountered previously: the idea of conception, and the idea of perception of things. This set of distinctions is crucial to this dissertation and the research it is based on. An appropriate starting point for examining the significance of conception, perception, rationality, and non—rationality lies with the model of C. G. Jung for categorizing people. The model is based on four functional typologies by which consciousness obtains its orientation to experience feeling, thinking, intuition, and sensing. Jung's definitions follow.

1. Feeling — "When I use the word 'feeling' in contrast to 'thinking,' I refer to judgment of value - for instance, agreeable or disagreeable, good, or bad, and so on. Feeling according to this definition is not an emotion."
2. Thinking – "...people who used their minds were those who 'thought' - that is, who applied their intellectual faculty in trying to adapt themselves to people and circumstances."
3. Intuition – "In so far as intuition is 'hunch,' it is not the product of a voluntary act; it is rather an involuntary event,

which depends upon different external or internal circumstances instead of an act of judgement."

4. Sensing – "(Like intuition, sensing is) more like a sense—perception, which is also an irrational event in so far as it depends essentially upon objective stimuli, which owe their existence to physical and not to mental causes."[104]

For Jung, feeling and thinking are dominantly rational functions used for "ordering" and are the product of voluntary mental events. Intuition and sensing, on the other hand, are dominantly non-rational functions used for "perceiving" and are the products of involuntary human events initiated by the physical world. Rational functions are triggered by the human mind, while non-rational functions are triggered by the environment. Both aspects are important for regulation in complex environments. Jung's summary of the four functions outlines the importance they could play in social regulation,

> Sensation (i.e., sense perception) tells you that something exists; <u>thinking</u> tells you what it is; <u>feeling</u> tells you whether it is agreeable or not; and <u>intuition</u> tells you whence it comes and where it is going.[105]

The appreciative mode of regulation developed within the dissertation rests on the integration of all four functions. Jung thought that everyone tended to emphasize one or the other of the functions. By including a wider set of individuals in a regulation process the conditions for accommodation of all four functions are enhanced. Grounding the mode of regulation in negotiation enhances the potential for interactivity between the functions. This should enhance the potential for integration of the functions. This takes the social regulation system well outside the traditional realm of limited human rationality. On the other hand, some individuals are strongly advocating movement towards a more realistic version of rationality

---

[104] C, G. Jung, 1964, p. 61.
[105] Jung, 1964, p. 61.

to better deal with processes like environmental deterioration. One example of this, which tended to typify a large section of the governmental thinking within the U.S. version of environmental protection, is offered by the proceedings of a Congressional Committee looking into regulatory problems in controlling environmental pollution. (Their discussions were dealing with obstacles to effective rationalization of problems in the environmental protection domain, e.g., economic, administrative, conceptual, etc.)

> Foremost among those obstacles is EPA's attitude toward its statutory responsibilities. Often it has been too timid... The range and strength of EPA's opposition suggests the need not only for EPA to pursue its mission more aggressively, but also for Congress to provide additional means by which EPA's activities and opposition can be monitored... Finally, EPA should adhere more closely to its statutory mandates.[106]

The individuals making the previous comment had been reacting to evidence given about dilemmas which were building up in the environmental protection regulation efforts to that date. One bit of evidence, presented from a Federal Court decision, which they had found especially distasteful was,

> Questions involving the environment are particularly prone to uncertainty. Technological man has altered his world in ways never experienced or anticipated. The health effects of such alterations are often unknown, sometimes unknowable. While a concerned Congress has passed legislation providing for protection of the public health against gross environmental modifications, the regulators entrusted with the enforcement of such laws have not thereby been

---

[106] "Federal Regulation and Regulatory Reform," an Oct. 1976 report of proceedings from the House Oversight Subcommittee, pp. 150—151.

endowed with a prescience that removes all doubt from their decision-making. [107]

The point of departure here is towards enlargement of the view of rationality, or failing in that attempt, to include, within a social regulation process, enough of the non—rational factors so that their characteristics can be accommodated. The limits of strict rationality are proving to be too restrictive to accommodate the multifaceted events we perceive in the empirical world. This is in accord with the idea of U Thant (1971) we must radically change our present systems which are based on rigid divisions, where "No rigid system, however well-established on a few sacrosanct principles, is able to cope with all the problems of our diverse, complex and constantly changing society."[108]

The conceptual environment, as used here, refers to Rapoport's (1974, p. 51) sense of the "symbolic environment." The perceptual environment in turn refers to his sense of the "physical environment." In the physical environment, man's actions are not that different from other animals' interactions with their environments.

> Overall, however, man's interaction with the physical environment differs only quantitatively, not qualitatively, from corresponding interactions of other animals with their environment. A house is but an elaborate nest, A superhighway is an improved cow path...

> The other environment, the symbolic one, has no analogue in the non-human world. There are no precursors among animals of epic poems, monuments, preferred stock, protest marches, confessions, astronomy, or astrology.

> Clearly, the degree to which man has been able to modify his physical environment (for better or for worse) is inti-

---

[107] Ibid., p. 149, originally from ETHYL CORP. v. EPA.
[108] Toronto, Canada, Globe and Mail, May 25, 1971.

mately related to certain features of his symbolic environment, to science, for example. The symbolic environment deserves careful examination as, perhaps, the most important determinant of the human condition.[109]

The conceptual (symbolic) environment contains the psychological landscape and the assorted structures which man places or finds there. Dostoevsky concentrated on this landscape so extensively that he hardly mentions the physical landscape. The perceptual environment in turn relies on the physical landscape, where man also places and identifies structures. Man-made and natural structures found in both landscapes are important to social regulation. A thesis is advanced here that current modes of regulation limit themselves to the physical environment, in that it is more tangible and implies more certainty, especially the man—made portions of it.

Dimensional Behavior: A Summary

0 Dimension – A Point Becoming Pointless
1 Dimension – A Line with Singularities at Each End
2 Dimension – Flatland, the Printed Word as Leadership
3 Dimension – Boxes, Cubic Outside Time, Hierarchies, Promissory Leadership
4 Dimension – Entropic, Outside Human Control, Negotiation Over Time via Diminished Leadership
5 Dimension – Different Kinds of Differences, Wisdom, Cosmic

Figure A Context for Understanding Climate Change Management

The importance of moving into the psychological environment is seen from the large role it plays as a factor inducing change, where

---

[109] Rapoport, 1974, p. 51.

to be viable a mode of regulation must be able to accommodate change.

Individuals and organizations expend considerable resources attempting to control natural phenomena and their dangers as posed upon mankind. Herein, is a thesis looking in the opposite direction. It examines current modes of regulation and concludes that they are not very competent in management of limiting the effect of human acts on nature. More important to humans is a related thesis that no mode of regulation can control the mostly autonomous relations from humans upon nature resulting in what we now call environmental deterioration. The ostensible purpose of this control has been to increase the opportunities to satisfy human needs. The thesis of this paper raises questions as to how well current modes of regulation can accomplish this. The paper also attempts to enlarge the purpose of regulation to include larger systems of life processes beyond man—made ordering.

> ... [It] is indeed true that we have created an ungovernable world, in which the natural order and a man—made order are blended as never before into a system which can be neither interpreted by natural nor governed by man-made laws.[110]

5. Regulation: Governance as False Hope

Two major pathways await humans in search of future success in relating to nature and the environment managed by nature. The challenge behind the work outlined herein is to discover evidence for which is timelier and offers more hope for beneficial change. 1) First is to institutionalize the means for humans to redefine self-interest via the dictates of environmental interest around different variables, variables beyond the limits of the Faustian Tragedy. 2) Second is to give more energy to the traditional manner of improving within the

---

[110] Vickers, 1970, p. 122

limits of Faustian negotiation but then lessen the consequences via broader and harsher punishment to those with the most losses piled highest around them. In other words, this would be expanded governance of the state via tougher regulations and harsher enforcement of the most noticeably bad humans.

The first approach is based on significant self-learning to achieve contextual appreciation. Humans tend to learn best via experiences that are most rude and pose the highest danger. This is of course a dilemma in that it always requires the threat of more time being needed than humans have available. We are not very good at finding leadership that can manage this dilemma and this time around the cost side of the dilemma is much more significant.

As such it is most likely that humans will turn to guaranteed failure in the second approach. Those with the resources can avoid, and the rest can ignore it. The expression used for this damage control, as found in the study, was that "More regulation is sort of acceptable, especially if my lawyers can help me get around it or delay its impact on me and my work." This is coming to be the essence of business school teachings in courses on "strategic management." This will worsen the situation in the mid-term but maybe can serve to make the first option more viable in the longer term. Perhaps the terror seen from results of those trained in a Harvard B-School model of strategic management can then give legitimation to something we might call "consequential management." This would be fundamentally different. It would require appreciation of consequences of results achievement in a manner that would enhance seeing the downside of those flawed results.

Relations between humans and nature will undoubtedly become rude, but hopefully will enhance learning in ways that can bring more rapid change to the necessary. Even now, in 1978, we see ominous environmental conditions approaching but little sign of needed response being apparent. Maybe we can only await the rudeness that allows us to better appreciate the differences between the good and bad, as well as the right and the wrong ways. Much of history shows a heavy bias towards reliance on the omnipresence of the bad to seek or create the good. The approach presented herein is quite different from the tradition of science in using causal thinking to set up analytic models to find the bad, via articulation of effects, then elimination of the cause. In this case we humans are the cause. Will we thus eliminate ourselves? Will punishment finally be found to make humans better? There is no record of it having worked previously.

Humans have long had trouble appreciating the good, defining, or even seeing it. Plato attempted to describe this in those trapped in his "Allegory of the Cave" seeing only two-dimensional shadows as reality. Goethe's depicted a similar sad state where Faust needed to be rich, intelligent, and accessible to beautiful others in the short-term. The price was an entity with no soul over the long term. A willingness to follow anyone who promises neg-entropy has long been the recipe to being a leader in business of government. All that is needed is for the top of the societal hierarchy to be strategic, to lie, and market nonsense then pretend access to the inaccessible.

Our accepted method of regulating others, and ourselves, has long been questionable based on its results. Regulation steeped in punishment only encourages those who are mean to become the managers of it and suggests that legal breakage need be done when no one is obviously looking. This includes shoplifting to environmental pollution control. There are clearly more effective ways to succeed in encouraging the good, ones that do not create dichotomies, dilemmas, polarization, and digital existence.

Criticizing and giving punishment for what has been done is generally ineffective in getting participants in society to do better, or even reflect on doing better. Many tests illustrate that to complement someone for doing good, without a regulatory requirement, shows how they are almost always encouraged to do good the next time. The law of the mean has long implied the opposite for strange reasons yet is often used as the core design of regulations. More specifically, if what was just done seems good, or better than the usual, then via "the law of the mean" we can pretend that the involved actor will become pushed towards the bad next time he acts. Continuing to follow such logic, we consistently see that if someone has done bad and are harshly criticized or punished for such, the statistical odds are that next time out he will do better than the mean. Sadly, lawyers and government actors often take this second route of relying on "next-time results" thinking to improve society. At a deeper level of statistics, we can see that such improvement almost always fails.

Perhaps the "waking up" option is most urgent, prior to encouraging right and/or discouraging wrong but that is not the subject herein. How best to help humans appreciate an approaching storm by educating them is important but not our subject. Besides, past research shows that humans tend to learn best via rude experiences in the beginning of the storm. Once it seems too late, humans can quickly respond. History illustrates how humans primarily respond via option b above with option a coming later as part of societal education. In most instances option b, encouraging humans to stop doing bad, involves governance with its structure resting on regulation. This has become the favored societal choice in modern times. As such, regulation is the focus herein as a problem-solving activity. This is not done with a sense of optimism that regulation can avert the ominous situation now approaching the conditions of life on earth but to argue that current approaches to regulation seem assured of failure. Something more appreciative of the problem faced and more robust in the human response may well be needed. This may be a different form of regulation or a shift towards option a, a broad encouragement of humans to consider the good and innovatively work towards it. It is hoped that an explicit failure of the traditional of regulation will redirect humans to experiment with option a. The normal long timetable for this approach can be greatly collapsed.

R.E.M.'s song, "Everybody Hurts," is one way to better visualize the content of this book, and thus understand humans driving around looking for the meaning to existence. They want to find some form of self to value. In the video of the song everyone stops on an expressway and sits while quietly reflecting on their situation. Then everyone exits their cars and begins walking with a knowing look on their faces, as if they finally have a place to which they want to go.

APPENDEX: DOORWAYS TO A FUTURE

2003: Hawk's Annotated Bibliography

David Hawk, a passer-by in life who has spent 30 years developing the upmost respect for NJIT students. The leadership of New Jersey Institute of Technology was not so great, as they seemed to have nowhere to go to, but the students, from relatively modest means, great experiences in negotiations with hell, and a sense of humor, were incredible people to learn from. All teachers who liked to teach that passed through NJIT before being dumped by leadership loved the students.

The following book list is dedicated to those students who helped compile the list and its annotations between 1981-2003. They took the titles and authors from Hawk lectures and publications where they loved to argue with all that was Hawk, thus they did their homework buying books. A past NJIT President of NJIT, and as a temporary Dean of Honors to make him eligible to be a president, was displeased with use of these books. To Hawk's boss he demanded Hawk be removed from teaching honor's students. He argued Hawk's teaching made things difficult for other professors in Honors, which had been Hawk's point. Not being able to remove Hawk from Honor's Teaching, he participated in the NJIT confiscated of a copy of most of these books claiming they were NJ State Property. Ha..ha. funny man, as you see upon reflection many leaders are funny men, except the consequences of their leadership are not fun or funny.

Hawk took many classes on international trips to meet companies he advised. The St. Petersburg's Art Museum, seen below, was a side trip to see the importance of 3-D in "Art Against Ideology," by Ernest Fisher. Such great works are doorways into other images of our world, images that can define your life.

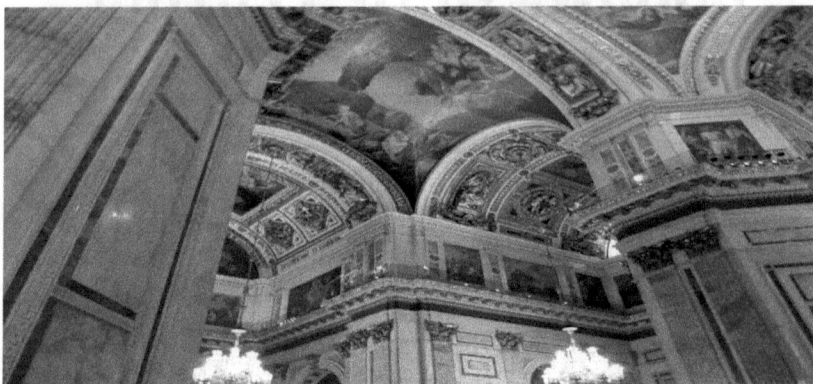

Once Euclid is Missing There is Hope.....

BOOKS: MORE THAN FURNITURE IN THE MIND

DAVID HAWK, PROFESSOR: SCHOOLS OF ARCHITECTURE & MANAGEMENT, NEW JERSEY INSTITUTE OF TECHNOLOGY

FEBRUARY 13, 2003

These books outline my history of ideas. I found them helpful to gaining access to life. I hope some prove to inspire you as they did me. Many qualify for membership in the great books of history library. I hope they lead you to look into other great books. These were helpful to my understanding of life and ways of living. Of course, reading is not everything, but it does allow access to almost everything. Herein you can gain access to inspiration in life as well as learning of those differences that make a difference in life. As Kurt Vonnegut put it many years ago:

> *"Hello babies. Welcome to Earth. It's hot in the summer and cold in the winter. Its round and wet and crowded. At the outside, babies, you've got about a hundred years here. There's only one rule that I know of babies—God damn it, you've got to be kind."*

— Kurt Vonnegut, *God Bless You, Mr. Rosewater*

My love of books came from my mother, a teacher of 2ⁿᵈ Grade students during her life. The love was enhanced by my high school principal without principles and teachers who could not teach via their banning me from all college preparatory courses in English, math, and the sciences, for defying their authority in life. I thus read about such subjects. Most of all I owe a great deal to my best friend in life, Gunnar Hedlund of the Stockholm School of Economics. After

277

meeting him in our first class in the Wharton School PhD program he took me aside and said, "Obviously you like books David, but as obvious is that that you have not read much, nor the best books." He took me directly to the Penn University bookstore and bought me six books to begin with. While I was teaching at the Stockholm School of Economics, I would compose a list of two hundred books to read each year. The Stockholm Library was just next door and the Institute of International Business he and I created came to be filled with students also loving books.

You might note that ideas in my lectures come from works of literature. They offered me a variety of reflections upon living, inspirations about life and ways to manage dangerous echoes from the past. I now have a 5,000-book collection in my Iowa home. Hopefully, this short list helps you gain expressions for that which you have long wanted access to but didn't know how to put it.

Some may not be an author's best work. I do not know. I found all of them to be insightful into what mattered to me at the time of reading them. I did not worry about their linguistic evaluation from experts in linguistics. They were "doorways" into an author's mind. Multiple books by a single author are encouraged in that they provide multiple doorways onto the same terrain, or even multiple terrains. I appreciated all of it, even the depressing enlightenment from those such as Ernst Fisher's in his 1966 writing. Therein he speculated on our future relative to an ever-expanding reliance on computers to interact with life.

"With increasing momentum, increasingly large masses of human beings, goods, arms, inventions, and technical achievements are moving towards a future whose face is veiled and whose body is a chimera, a machine with an archangel's wings, a fantastically rapid alternation of ultra-light and deep, terrible night. The more precisely computers calculate this future, the less we can face the incalculable. The more closely we predict what will happen in twenty years' time, the more unexpected are the events of today. We are lost in a perfectly constructed maze of facts, dates, and information. Ariadne's threat has multiplied a hundred-fold; we do not know which one we should follow, and stumble from one dead-end into another. A plethora of means has devoured the end." *Art Against Ideology*, P. 37.

Another close friend, and mentor, Hasan Ozbekhan, once commented on the art of book writing. He had been talking about our mutual friend, Russell Ackoff, who had written 20+ books. Hasan hesitated in writing his first by pointing out that there already seemed to be too much truth out there for consumption by humans. He went on to comment: "David, in each person there is one book. If we are lucky, we get that book out prior to our death. If our friends are unlucky, we rewrite that book twenty times over and expect them to read it all." I miss Hasan.

We might say that we are all engaged in a lifelong search to find those differences that make a difference. A Gregory Bateson idea it came to be crucial to understanding why human say what they do, then do something else. Such ideas raise amazing insights as finding the amazing people and seeing humor in the non-so-amazing kind, usually occupied by leaders that couldn't.

Crucial to me was understanding of a) *thermodynamic entropy*, b) the *Faustian Tragedy*, and c) *Being nice*.

ENTROPY: This idea emphasizes a fundamental importance in **context** to evaluate our human actions, actions they may bring you to meet climate change consequences. Context, for entropic purposes, as defined by industrialization is where humans meet fulfillment of human needs. In a context humans search for a life with meaningful wants and ways to meet them. Thus, the human project becomes an economic struggle with and against things, usually yet to be defined. AI proposes as a new dawn with new beginnings in finding and meeting needs. AI is neither true, natural nor viable, but we will eagerly embrace it as continuation of the industrialization path they used to support who they thought they were.

Moving from industrialization to "post-industrialized" is insignificant. It's mostly a marketing of continuation of mechanistic themes. As we spend more time in front of our machines there is little sign of our returning to the natural any time soon. That is a pity. As a basis to our life this industrial model brings with it much environmental deterioration. In twenty years we will see how this becomes climate change with quite expensive consequences. None-the-less, such seems like the essence of being human in our economic thinking and desires. Maybe we can't expect much more. Sorry. To better understand this look into that most fundamental of laws of the universe, "**the second law of thermodynamics.**" We know it is important in that it is one of the most ignored laws in university education in engineering and business. It appears as against both. **The first law** allows for some optimism; thus, it is easily accepted by humans. The **second law**, the entropy law, is more avoided as it become more relevant. Sadly, it governs our reality more than any other law. In weaker schools, it is completely ignored. In stronger schools, it is carefully toned down or put on a shelf to be seen but not examined.

Sometimes referenced, and not examined, it explains life expirations. In classes where you are encouraged to create immortality projects, why become confused in finding the existence of entropy, thus mortality? The US Congress went so far as to not allow patens on Neg-Entropy discoveries in the 1930's, in that they thought there would be a rush of them to get out from the depression. Seemingly the Congressmen has not been informed that neg-entropy can't exist.

The wise, e.g., Einstein, cautioned us to avoid those who argue for discovery of negative entropy to support human affairs. Such humans are either out to cheat you, or too stupid to trust. Hawking went deeper, although a bit more poetic, in agreeing with Einstein about the importance of the entropy law relative to human quality.

> "The human race is just a chemical scum on a moderate-sized planet, orbiting around a very average star in the outer suburb of one among a hundred billion galaxies. We are so insignificant that I can't believe the whole universe

exists for our benefit. That would be like saying that you would disappear if I closed my eyes." — Stephen Hawking in "Reality on the Rocks" TV series (AP)

If designers took entropy into consideration, via design, then resulting products and processes would be quite different. Via such thinking humans might even avoid climate change consequences. Oh well, so much for that dream.

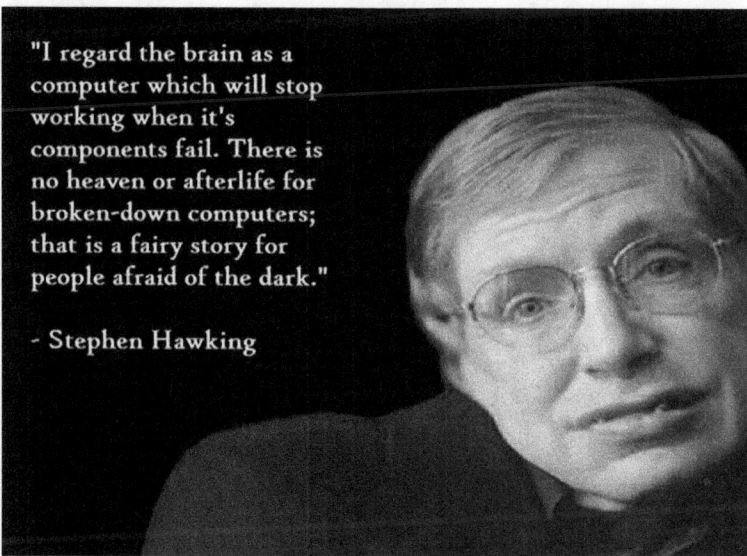

"I regard the brain as a computer which will stop working when it's components fail. There is no heaven or afterlife for broken-down computers; that is a fairy story for people afraid of the dark."

- Stephen Hawking

THE FAUSTIAN TRAGEDY: The second item brought up in every course I would teach is ethics. This I believe is fundamental to any deep understanding of the human project. Just now we are a project that is creating a deteriorated context, i.e., via our lives we generate environmental deterioration. We do this via bargaining. This is the essence of Goethe's 1781 Faustian Tragedy, Parts I and II. The Faustian character emerged in 1550 around Martin Luther and his obvious shortcomings. The story of Faust, as the symbol of humans wanting to sell their souls to their devils, reached a low point in the 1945 story from Paul Valery. He described how all humans were out to sell their souls, and for any price, but the devil who normally negotiated the price had gone into hiding to seek protection from this unmanageable evil called humans.

> Another way to work through the ethical dilemma humans face daily is to think about the conception of there being **both plus more.** In this system of thought all conflicts, dilemmas, contradictions, irrelevant differences, and made-up problems are sent to where they belong in the cosmic scheme. The "more" becomes a third candidate in the dilemma, one offering hope. It includes and operates above the limitations of the irresolvable two. As such, any arguments created in economics, politics, religions, and relations to life can be appreciated, laughed at and perhaps temporarily resolved by raising them to a higher level. There, the "more" matters most and includes the two. The wars behind capitalism and communism, Christians and Muslims, men and women, dogs and cats are shifted into another frame. Including the weaknesses and strengths of both provides a platform, not an answer. Addressing climate change by seeing how both capitalism and communism contribute to it equally sets the stage to find the "more." Consequences from climate change, such as no national boundaries remaining due to mass migration, will introduce the importance of the more. The "more," especially as seen in ethics, is accessible when we feel then begin to see "it's too late."

Once it's too late those in charge of creating the mess go underground to save their slippery skins. This provides a stage to begin to allow non-strategic, ethical behavior to emerge in those left. The danger then is that once a viable world is again discovered the slime has a way of leaving their shelters and moving back into the system. This can be seen in many organizations, including universities, churches, families, and companies. It is worth your time to contemplate the "more." There is much to be discovered therein. I trust you see hope in ethics as more. If not then you are welcome to become a member of the darker side.

The darker side? What is that? My 1979 dissertation at the Wharton School of Business dealt with aspects of the darker side in human affairs. It was based on one of the first research studies into the emergence of something called climate change and discovered the profound role of US trained lawyers in insuring we would not stop it in a timely manner. The importance of suspending ethics in arriving at a "legalese" based regulatory system was carefully documented alongside evidence of how it tends to increase in environmental pollution. Many firms with similar production facilities in many different nations were used as the test base. The production and ownership were fixed, and the regulatory system was variable. My Chair, Russell Ackoff said the three volumes of research behind the work were the best PhD document he had ever seen and illustrated why he had started the PhD program.

By 2020 the vision of the consequences of our acts will be clear enough so that our children will begin to be very unhappy with us. The feelings of our grandchildren will undoubtedly be fearsome. They will not understand how we could have been as we now are. Now, in 2003 you have probably not heard much about a 19th Century, Newton-based approach to industrialization, all managed via 18th Century ideas of leadership. You will hear more in the future in terms of how it led to climate change, or whatever the great consequence of small results will come to be called. Until 2020 you will focus of your careers and your chances to find and buy life. In 2020 you may suddenly rethink what you thought was leadership in society. You may then come to consider the idea that it was mostly leadershit. So sorry. Maybe you can fix it?

Many subjects are on the following book list. You should be skeptical of all subject matter categorizations, and perhaps even all subjects. If you find a hierarchy of importance in categories, you have missed the point. Subject matters are used to help organize what is seen as a complex world, but you will pay for that view. Categories are artificial and often denote dead ends, especially if you organize your life around them. Libraries organize books into academic disciplines as they don't know what else to do. The subject you will take from school relative to what subjects you were taught in schools, will be profoundly different. This is good. Avoid notions that things are complicated. It usually means someone has a hierarchy in mind, where they oversee it.

Complexity of phenomena, like life, is only an excuse to not see it then to segment it into categories that are disassociated from each other and reality, thus losing the systemic connections that are the key to knowing life. All this is done in the name of logical understanding or learning to rely on unaided rationality to find meaning in meaninglessness. The cost to this pathway to understanding can be fatal to your understanding. Complexity is to be embraced and untangled, not praised, avoided, or buried under categories and subject labels.

Once you concentrate on the connections between parts you no longer see parts. Complexity is generally restricted to the eye of the beholder, and on closer inspection in not in what is being viewed. Normal academic approach generally presupposes subjects to be sacrosanct. You might note that nature shows little respect for what humans believe to be true, such as how humans carve up their world to make sense of it. Outside academia the world progresses by changing or avoiding categories. Shakespearean plays are good at pointing to this infinite pattern.

Systems of living order have little respect for humanly designed stage sets composed of academic, economic, or dramatic furniture. How humans come to relate to their planet, to other humans, then finally to their selves is what matters to life. Yes, we can change nature, but nature will then change us and the circumstances that define us. The consequences of industrialization and how it changes our water, land and air and the climate is becoming omnipresent to life, death and the meanings presented to us in between. Some of the works found herein address overriding concerns for our species but offer stories well beyond Shakespeare and his camp followers. Science provides brief glimpses into the limits of the human belief systems but offers no systematic picture of meaning. That seems to await our cumulative impacts on our environment since industrialization began its mechanical process. Seems the machine might be done by 2050. The climate stability needs for life are incompatible with the cumulative consequences of our industrial results. Pity.

Aspects of understanding via doorways into the psychological, social, and natural worlds are suggested in the headings that will follow. Please note that as you encounter the content of the actual books you see how the lines between disciplines fade allowing more relevant and significant differences and questions to arise. For example, the historic differences between art and science are soon replaced by integrations of the best aspects and talents of art and science, all to better understand human limits and conditions of existence.

If it helps you might reflect on the well-known Plato Allegory of the Cave. It offers a simple and clear doorway into the meaning of limits to human understanding of context and the role of humans in changing that context. In Plato's metaphor undated we see how he only allowed the 1% who were richest in society to escape the limits of the cave. They were allowed to follow the cracks that first allowed the light into the cave designed and maintained by them. It is worth noting that the escapees from the cave did choose to return to their leadership role in the seeming comfort of the cave's darkness and republicanisms. They commented that the light outside was too bright. The cracks continue to grow in the cave and at some point, all humans will need to leave its dark security. Democracy and democrats do not offer any sanctuary if education is as it is.

You may discover more in common, than in difference, between many of the books, their subjects, and the qualities of their writings. It is worthwhile to consider what they all hold in common. Perhaps you will even come to entertain the very strange notion in all good writing and the worthy human concern that drives the will to express. All expression seems to seek that same common statement, a statement humans will never express. We do not know that question, nor are able to state it but we should not stop trying to express it. Life is a process of wondering about, wandering around and tentatively discovering the nature of that question. Perhaps you may find a way to go beyond all the limitations in the books presented herein to state the ultimate human question(s). I don't know.

These books are on the shelves in my office. You may come look through them, touch and smell them, etc. When you feel a need to understand the context in which you live these give different perspectives on the same phenomenon: your life. Use them well.

NOTE in 2023: All these books were impounded in 2011 by NJIT President Altenkirch as "state property." I never saw them again. He was not known for his passion for reading thus there must have been another reason in his mind? An associate dean said they were probably burnt, as they upset leadership of NJIT so very much. I wonder why? Pity.)

I. AN INTRODUCTION TO IT ALL... (What is "it"?)

A. *At the Edge of History*, William Irwin Thompson, 1971.

"The technology of our industrial civilization has reached a peak in putting a man on the moon, but as the ancients knew, the peak is also the moment of descent. Before we ascend the next peak to Mars there is a very dark valley waiting beneath us, and, poetically enough, its darkness is made up of just those things our civilization did in order to succeed."

B. *Toward a History of Needs*, Ivan Illich, 1977.

"Wherever the shadow of economic growth touches us we are left useless unless employed on a job or engaged in consumption; the attempt to build a house or set a bone outside the control of certified specialists appears as anarchic conceit. We lose sight of our resources, lose control over the environmental conditions which make these resources applicable, lose taste for self-reliant coping with challenges from without and anxiety from within." (Also read this author's fundamental work: "The Disabling Professions." Contemporary professional training, as we have come to worship it and have our children aspire to it, was initiated via Hitler to keep students, and society from learning to much about connections and context, thus asking "why?")

C. *Player Piano,* Kurt Vonnegut, Jr. 1951. For those who like music, anti-music, and other related difficulties in knowing what is going on.

D. *Stand on Zanzibar,* John Brunner, 1968. "Negro -Member of a subgroup of the human race who hails, or whose ancestors hailed, from a chunk of land nicknamed -not by its residents -Africa. Superior to the Caucasian in that the Negroes did not invent nuclear weapons, the automobile, Christianity, nerve gas, the concentration camp, military epidemics, or the megalopolis."

E. *The Wisdom of Insecurity,* Alan Watts, 1951. Interesting, soft...and more.

F. *Celebrations of Life,* Rene Dubos, 1981. "The word 'life' denotes not what living organisms are made of, but what they do. Observations and scientific studies have provided much knowledge about living creatures and especially human beings ...but this biological knowl-edge does not reveal how life is experienced." From his last book. If interested, look into: *The mirage of Health, A God within, So Human an Animal and The Wooing of the Earth.*

G. *Denial of Death,* Ernest Becker, 1974. The prospect of death, Dr. Johnson said, wonderfully concentrates the mind. The main thesis of this book is that it does much more than that: the idea of death, the fear of it, haunts the human animal like nothing else; it is a main-spring of human activity -activity designed largely to avoid the fatal-ity of death, to overcome it by denying in some way that it is the final destiny for man. A book about humans developing a need to invent and manage "immortality projects" to deny their mortality in life. Becker claims these "projects" are the base camp of much evil revealed to the world. He was writing the follow-up book on how to "*Escape from Evil*" when he too died.

H. *The Complete Traveller in Black,* John Brunner, 1986. 'As you wish, so be it,' declares the traveler in black, and the forces of the universe that bend to his will. The spoken words of the wisher come to be, but the results are scarcely what the wisher really desired. Instead, the results help the world achieve order and vanquish human chaos. This is a chronicle of the beginning of the world as we know it -the world of order and reason -a world partly fashioned by the enigmatic traveler in black. Only the traveler works knowingly on the side of order and reason. His enemies, at first, are numerous, until they eliminate themselves by realizing their own wishes.

I. *The Shockwave Rider*, John Brunner, 1975. This introduces many of the terms later used by computer hackers, as well as the terms used to frame what will become the lost world of big data. A must read for those interested in to where we will be via data collection religions in 2020 and beyond. Those interested in the limits of Artificial Intelligence and how it will sadly replace declining Human Intelligence will be shocked at the wisdom of Brunner. To see hope there remains the world of Natural Intelligence but we have less access to nature with time. We file it under the supernatural and return to problems with logic, such as why if one man can accomplish a work task in 60 seconds why the hell can't we manage to get sixty men complete it in 1 second? That is what MBA programs are all about via their combining the limits of operations research to human resource management thereby arriving at eviler than what can be counted in either alone.

I. *Looking Glass Universe,* John P. Briggs, 1984. A fascinating look into the basis of the modern revolution in physics, mathematics, chemistry, biology, and neurophysiology, as well as the ideas of the scientists whose startling new theories change our understanding of how the universe works.

J. *Civilization & Capitalism: 15th-18th Century,* Fernand Braudel: These three volumes encourage the reader to appreciate and perhaps even like history. Much different than what you find reading usually accepted American historians.

- Volume 1 -The Structures of Everyday Life
- Volume 2 -The Wheels of Commerce
- Volume 3 -The Perspective of the World

II. ON ART, ARCHITECTURE, PLANNING, DESIGN, OTHER HUMANISTIC AND/ OR ARTIFICIAL INTERVENTIONS...

A. *Zen and the Art of Motorcycle Maintenance,* Robert Pirsig, 1974. One of the best books written on the nature of quality and the quality of nature.

And what is good, Phaedrus

And what is not good - Need we ask anyone to tell us these things?

B. The *City* in *History,* Lewis Mumford, 1933. A good overview to concepts of from where the urban condition comes, and to where it seems to go.

C. Art *Against Ideology,* Ernst Fischer, 1966. New ideas opposing petrified ideologies cause unrest, stimulate opposition, eventually grip the masses, and turn into actual power. ...In all ideologies ideas are arrested so that they become 'idees fixes,' immovable supports of a class, a system, a ruling group. What is lost is the movement of the idea, therefore its dialectic and therefore its reality. The idea is placed in a coffin of dogma. Ideologies are fortresses. Ideas operate in open territory, measure their forces in direct combat, test one another, learn through contradiction, and then come home enriched by experience...

D. *Flatland,* Edwin Abbott, 1888. I call our world flatland, not because we call it so, but to make its nature clearer to you, my happy readers, who are privileged to live in space.

Imagine a vast sheet of paper on which Straight Lines, Triangles, Squares, Pentagons, Hexagons, and other figures, instead of remaining fixed in their places, move freely about, on or in the surface, but without the power of rising above or sinking below it, very much like shadows – only hard and with luminous edges - and you will then have a pretty correct notion of my country and countrymen.

E. *File Under Architecture,* Herbert Muschamp, 1974. I'm an architect who has neither designed nor built any buildings nor has the inclination to do so. I call myself an architect purely out of the comic conceit which is all that remains of the Western architectural tradition. Buildings have such short life spans nowadays, and few bother to look at them anyway.

F. *Tomorrow* is Our *Permanent Address,* John and Nancy Jack Todd, 1980. A bio-shelter is one actualization of an emerging theory of design that is based on natural systems, of a bio-technic approach to the problems of human sustenance.

G. *Design of Cities,* Edmund Bacon, 1969. As good a book on planning and city-making as you will find, written by as good a man as you will find, who worried about goodness in cities and the people who built and occupy them. He was a friend. I was allowed to be his teaching assistant.

H. *Poems and Prophecies,* William Blake, 1927. To see a World in a Grain of Sand And a Heaven in a Wild Flower, Hold Infinity in the palm of your hand And Eternity in an hour.

If you want to know more about Blake's work and its implications in science and philosophy see Donald Ault's *Visionary Physics: Blake's Response to Newton,* 1974 and David Erdman's *Blake: Prophet Against*

Empire, 1954. To go even deeper, and broader, into understanding the present look into the science of holography, which are the children of Blake's sandy ancestor.

I. *Steps to an Ecology of Mind,* Gregory Bateson, 1972. (Ballantine edition.) Metalogue, i.e., why things have outlines?

> Daughter: Daddy, why do things have outlines?
> Father: Do they? I don't know. What sort of things do you
>   mean?
> D: I mean when I draw things, why do they have outlines?
> F: Well, what about other sorts of things -a flock of sheep?
>   or a conversation? Do they have outlines?
> D: Don't be silly. I can't draw a conversation. I mean *things?*
> F: Yes -I was trying to find out just what you meant. Do
>   you mean "Why do we give things outlines when we
>   draw them?" or do you mean that the things *have*
>   outlines whether we draw them or not?
> D: I don't know, Daddy. You tell me. What do I Mean?
> F: I don't know, my dear. There was a very angry artist
>   once (Blake) who scribbled all sorts of things down,
>   and after he was dead they looked in his books and
>   in one place they found he'd written 'Wise men
>   see outlines and therefore they draw them' but in
>   another place he'd written 'Mad men see outlines
>   and therefore they draw them.'

Bateson's thought about the human future: "Mankind is going to have to learn how to make himself more predictable; otherwise the machines are going to become angry and kill him."

J. *Alice's Adventures in Wonderland,* Lewis Carroll, 1865. A good beginning, and, perhaps even the ending story for the human tragedy. A wonderful guidebook to international business theory during the 1990s, but not thereafter. Other themes now rule business. The work is related to but perhaps deeper than the theme of "The Wizard of Oz." The illustrator of the Wizard of Oz, Mr. O'Neil, owned and lived at my Mt. Olive horse farm for many years. Please come visit as you will see how the architecture and nature inspired his work.

K. *Architects' Data* Neufert, 1990. If you must think in the Germany way, and some of you must, then this is the essence of it for those believe they are architects. It is organized in the best of the 20th Century German tradition. Warning: read Bateson first to get a sense of what "un-aided consciousness" will do for and to you, so that this 20th Century data dump will be more useful, and funny.

L. *The Castle,* Kafka 1926. It was late in the evening when K. arrived. The village was deep in snow. The Castle hill was hidden, veiled in mist and darkness, nor was there even a glimmer of light to show that a castle was there. On the wooden bridge leading from the main road to the village, K. stood for a long time gazing into the illusory empties.

M. *Building the Unfinished,* Lars Lerup, 1977. Extraordinarily pro-architecture and anti-architect as students are currently taught to be in Schools of Architecture. Points out that the best in life and human experience is never finished but always evolving towards a greater end then humans envision. Good students seem to love this book, prior to transferring to other subjects that are more fluid. Herein is demonstrated the underlying problem in current architectural schools, and a source of much teacher frustration:

"It is very hard to kill a talent."

III. PHILOSOPHY, SOME WESTERN, SOME EASTERN, AND SOME FROM FRAGMENTS IN THE HUMAN SOUL

A. *The Story of Philosophy*, Will Durant 1926. A sourcebook on Western philosophy, covering approximately twenty of the most noted philosophers in the Western world of thought.

B. *The Wisdom of Lao-Tze,* Modern Library Edition Translation 1949. A much simpler approach to the search for truth, consisting of only 5,000 words.

C. *Methods of Inquiry* Churchman and Ackoff, 1950. A return to the subject matter of Durant's book but with a clear taste of the need for much more than what is available within the limits of rational thought. An introduction and overview of the relations between philosophy and scientific methods, as it has developed during the past 2,000 years in the West. An excellent sourcebook for a Management Ph.D. It is especially for those interesting in the philosophy of science, but quite difficult to locate.

D. *The Meeting of the East and West* C.F. Northrup. A good attempt at combining the meaning of differences between Eastern and Western thought, relative to current situations and emergent international issues. Also look to C.P. Snows "Two Cultures" for an elaboration on this concern, but of course with a fundamental difference of what the cultures represent.

E. *A Sourcebook in Chinese Philosophy,* Wing-tsit Chan, 1963. An introduction to those who wish to find a basis for comparing Eastern and Western thinking processes. Helpful to both sides of the relationship, but not helpful to seeing there is one nor finding a path to the "third" way.

F. *The Secret of the Golden Flower,* Richard Wilhelm, 1931. For those who like flowers...and other beautiful things in life.

G. *Philosophy in a New Key,* Susanne Langer, 1942. An excellent study in the importance of symbolism of reason, rite, and art. Important to development of contemporary forms of meaning, thought and philosophy. Also important to micro-processor and computer language developments. From reading this it become interesting to see how studiously those now doing it use her terms but leave out her recommendations on inclusion of rite and art in information technology. Too bad.

> "There are relatively few people today who are born to an environment, which gives them spiritual support. Only persons of some imagination and effective intelligence can picture such an environment and deliberately seek it. They are the few who feel drawn to some realm of reality feel drawn to some realm of reality which contains their ultimate life-symbols and dictates activities which may acquire ritual value...Any man who loves his calling loves it for more than its use; he loves it because it seems to have meaning."(p. 288)

H. *Ch'i: A Neo-Taoist Approach to Life,* RGH Siu, 1974.

Musing is delightful freedom. No one claims the jurisdiction, sets the rules, or challenges the outcome. You can muse at any time, in any place, and under any circumstance. Never does it dip into the pits of evil. It ennobles and enlightens and suffuses as with a quiet joy. Free of logic. Carefree of consensus. Free and carefree in essence. It's a shame that MBA students, via Maslow's Hierarchy of Needs, are instructed how to find and fire people doing this to improve what the Economist worships as "productivity."

IV. SCIENCES

A. *One Two Three...Infinity,* George Gamow, 1947.

...of atoms, stars, and nebulae, of entropy and genes; and whether one can bend space, and why the rocket shrinks. And indeed, in this book we are going to discuss all these topics, and also many others of equal interest.

B. *The ABC of Relativity,* Bertrand Russell, 1959. (Simply fun)

Everybody knows that Einstein did something astonishing, but very few people know exactly what is was that he did. It is generally recognized that he revolutionized our conception of the physical world, but the new conceptions are wrapped up in mathematical technicalities.

C. *The Structure of Scientific Revolutions,* Thomas Kuhn, 1962. (More serious)

Scientific knowledge, life, language, is intrinsically the common property of a group or else nothing at all. To understand it we shall need to know the special circumstances of the groups that create and use it. Argues for the fluid but does so in a way that the fixed have come to use him to deter the fluid.

D. *Scientific Method,* Russell Ackoff, 1962. (Much more serious)

The book is definitely slanted to the decision maker, the man of affairs, the manipulator of men, machines and resources...However, the bulk of this book is not written from the point of view of the humanities. The title does not say this. Therefore, the preface should say it in no uncertain terms, namely, that scientific method is treated here from a certain point of view, where the point of departure is a problem defined in what to do terms. (Anatol Rapoport's preface to the book.)

E. *Against Method,* Feyerabend, 1962. (An alternative)

Claiming that anarchism must now replace rationalism in the theory of knowledge, Feyerabend argues that intellectual progress can only be achieved by stressing the creativity and wishes of the scientist rather than the method and authority of science. In the later half of the book he examines Popper's 'critical rationalism' and the attempt by Lakatos to construct a methodology, which allows the scientist his freedom without threatening scientific 'law and order.' Rejecting both attempts to shore up rationalism, he looks forward to the 'withering away of reason' and maintains that 'the only principle which does not inhibit progress is anything goes.'

F. *The Art of Scientific Investigation,* W. Beveridge, 1950.

G. *Godel's Proof,* Ernest Nagel and James Newman, 1958.

H. *Godel, Escher, Bach,* Douglas Hofstadter, 1979.

I. *Darwin and the Mysterious Mr. X,* Loren Eiseley, 1979. J. *The Fourth Dimension,* Rudy Rucker, 1984.

K. *Chaos: Making a New Science,* James Gleick, 1987.

> Over the last decade, physicists, biologists, astronomers, and economists have created a new way of understanding the growth of complexity in nature. This new science, called chaos, offers a way of seeing order and pattern where formerly only the random, the erratic, the unpredictable -in short, the chaotic -had been observed. In the words of Douglas Hofstadter, 'It turns out that an Erie type of chaos can lurk just behind a facade of order -and yet, deep inside the chaos lurks an even eerier type of order.

L. *Linked: The New Science of Networks,* Albert-Laszlo Barabasi, Cambridge, Ma.: Perseus Publishing, 2002. Good stuff.

M. *The Gifts of Athena: Historical Origins of the Knowledge Economy,* Joel Mokyr, And Princeton, NJ: Princeton University Press, 2002.

N. *The End of Science*, John Horgan, New York: Addison-Wesley Publishing, 1996. A stunningly interesting book on how science becomes a religion, therefore limiting to the human intellect via projects that should not be accomplished.

V. SYSTEMS APPROACHES TO PROBLEM SOLVING

A. *The Systems Approach and Its Enemies,* C. West Churchman, 1979.

You first might what to look at Churchman's 1966 book, *The Systems Approach*.

B. *Redesigning the Future,* Russell Ackoff, 1974. An important book that shows how an eminent social scientist turned the comer from the quantitative towards the qualitative dimension of problem solving. This was his penance for having written "On Purposeful Systems."

C. *Systems Thinking,* F.E. Emery, 1969. A basic book for anyone interested in use of systems approaches in organizations.

D. *Foundations for a Science of Personality,* Andras Angyal, 1941. Perhaps the most basic book in the 20th Century on ideas and challenges called for development of systems thinking. For example, this book introduces the notion that as a system reaches its limits 'the parts assume the whole.' What this means has long been a challenge in systems. With holography we now have a much better physical model of what it means, but not yet a psychological or research model.

E. *Change,* Paul Watslawick, John Weakland, and Richard Fisch, 1974. This book deals with the age-old questions of persistence and change in human affairs. More particularly, it is concerned with how problems arise and are perpetuated in some instances and resolved in others. It examines how, paradoxically, common sense and logical

approaches often fail and in doing so compound an existing problem, while seemingly 'illogical' and 'unreasonable' actions succeed in
producing the desired change.

F. *Ackoff's Best*, Russell L. Ackoff, New York: John Wiley and Sons,
1999.

VI. THE POLITICS OF HUMANKIND, NOT KIND HUMANS

A. *The New Leviathan,* RG Collingwood, 1942.

What is Man?

Before beginning to answer the question, we must know why it is
asked. It is asked, because we are beginning an inquiry into civilization, and the revolt against it which is the most conspicuous thing
going on at the present time.

B. *Twilight of Authority,* Robert Nisbet, 1975.

I believe the single most remarkable fact at the present time in the
West is neither technological nor economic, but political: the waning
of the historic political community, the widening sense of the obso-
lescence of politics as a civilized pursuit, even as a habit of mind.

C. *Anarchism,* George Woodcock, 1962.

A history of libertarian ideals and movements.

D. *Mutual Aid,* Peter Kropotkin, 1918.

E. *Government and the Mind,* Joseph Tussman, 1977.

An overreaction of the possibilities of anarchism?

VII. THE ECONOMICS OF HUMANKIND

A. *The Ultimate Resource,* Julian Simon, 1981.

Have a strong stomach with you on this trip...

"Is there a natural resource problem? Certainly, there is -just as there has always been. The problem is that natural resources are scarce, in the sense that it costs us labor and capital to get them, though we would prefer to get them for free.

Are we now "entering an age of scarcity"? You can see anything you like in a crystal ball. But almost without exception, the best data -the long-run economic indicators -suggest precisely the opposite. The relevant measures of scarcity -the costs of natural resources in human labor, and their price relative to wages and to other goods -all suggest that natural resources have been becoming less scarce over the long run, right up to the present."

B. *The Entropy Law and the Economic Process,* Nicholas Georgescu-Roegen, 1971.

An alternative to the book listed in A, for those with intelligence and concern for people who need, believe in, and even read works such as the one of Simon.

VIII. THE POTENTIALS OF HUMANS

A. *The Human Side of Enterprise,* Douglas McGregor, 1960.

The book presents two radically different attitudes towards management; one is technical in orientation and looks to humans as a physical resource participating in the total machine called production. The other is humanistic in outlook and looks into the humanistic requirements in the work setting that are psychological, as well as physical and technical. (Those teaching HR in MBA programs would never understand this thesis. Perhaps that lack is the entry requirement for them to enter the sad world of HRM?)

B. *The Human Use of Human Beings,* Norbert Wiener, 1956.

A rather optimistic book on the science of cybernetics and its role in improving the human condition. Several of the underlying presumptions about a 'post-industrial' society are found in this early work. Reading this along with Gregory Bateson's work provides a beginning and ending to cybernetics, then a warning about the limits of AI, but no one is listening. Avoid Cybernetics and schools that praise it. The best programs do so, see how information technology is taught in Asia for a non-cybernetic approach.

C. *Towards a Social Ecology,* Emery and Trist, 1973.

Difficult but well worth the reading effort. It outlines the underlying value differences the make up the current world and a more beneficial world that ought to be.

D. *The Act of Creation,* Arthur Koestler, 1964. Great book.

E. *Mind, Discovering the,* Walter Kaufmann, 1980. Unparalleled work on the mind.

- Volume I, Goethe, Kant and Hegel
- Volume II, Nietzsche, Heidegger, and Buber
- Volume III, Freud versus Adler and Jung

IX. THE DARKER SIDE OF HUMANS

A. *The Mountain People,* Colin Turnbull, 1972. Tough stuff about the weak.

B. *The Arrogance of Humanism,* David Ehrenfeld, 1978. Tough stuff against the entire human project and how the weaker people, spiritually, tend to be allowed to lead it.

C. *Social Darwinism,* Robert Bannister, 1979. From this begins understanding of what 19th Century humans did, then what 20th Century humans do and what 21st Century humans want to do. This is a sad thesis but reliance on it is essential to understanding the thinking of the misnamed conservatives in American society. Via their belief in "survival of the fattest" they care most for the bankers, not those who provide the goods and services. This attitude provides a pathway to complete hopelessness.

D. *Journey to the End of the Night* 1934 & *Death on the Installment Plan,* 1952, Louis-Ferdinand Celine. Warning, this is not an easy read for the soul. Two of my favorites

E. *Billiards at Halfpast Nine: Builders and Destroyers,* Heinrich Boll. Another kind of poetic statement on the human condition in that it's a story about a son who is expected to destroy, during a wartime offensive, the church that his father had created.

F. *The Inner-City Mother Goose,* Eve Merriam, 1969. There was a crooked man. And he did very well.

G. *The Heart of a Dog,* 1925 and *The Master and Margarita,* 1938, Mikhail Bulgakov The title says it all.

H. *Briefing for a Descent into Hell,* Doris Lessing, 1972.

Again, the title says it all, and not what you would call optimistic.

X. TO FIND A WAY OUT FROM IX.

A. Carlos Castaneda:

- *The Teachings of Don Juan*
- *A Separate Reality*
- *Journey to Extlan*
- *Tales of Power.*

B. Walter Kaufman (He also did the previously listed "mind" set.)
- *The Future of the Humanities,* 1977.
- *Without Guilt and Justice,* 1973.
- *Tragedy and Philosophy,* 1968.

C. Herman Hesse
- *Demian*
- *Steppenwolf*
- *Magister Ludi*

D. John Dos Passos
- *The 42nd Parallel.*
- *The Big Money*
- *Nineteen Nineteen*

E. Goethe
- *The Sorrow of Young Walter*
- *Faust: Part I*
- *Faust: Part II*

F. Fydor Dostoyevsky
- *Crime and punishment*
- *The Idiot*
- *The Brothers Karamazov*

G. Erving Goffman
- *Asylums*
- *Frame Analysis*
- *The Presentation of Self in Everyday Life*

H. *The phenomenon of Man,* Teilhard de Chardin, 1954.

I. The I Ching or Book of Changes, Richard Wilhelm translation, 1951.

J. *Walden* & *Other Writings*, Henry David Thoreau, 1937.

K. *Mutual Aid*, Peter Kropotkin, 1914.

Best of luck in your journies through life.
If in doubt, be nice...

www.ingramcontent.com/pod-product-compliance
Lightning Source LLC
Chambersburg PA
CBHW062116020426
42335CB00013B/985